Complementary&
Alternative Medicine
in Breastfeeding Therapy

Nikki Lee, RN, BSN, MS, IBCLC, CCE, CIMI, ANLC, CST (Appl. Cert.)

© Copyright 2011

Hale Publishing, L.P.

Complementary and Alternative Medicine in Breastfeeding Therapy

Nikki Lee, RN, MS, IBCLC, CCE, CIMI, ANLC, CST (Appl. Cert.)

Hale Publishing, L.P.
1712 N. Forest St.
Amarillo, TX 79106-7017
806-376-9900
800-378-1317
www.iBreastfeeding.com
www.halepublishing.com

Library of Congress Control Number: 2011925701

ISBN-13: 978-0-9833075-5-6

Printing and Binding: Friesens
Printed in Canada

Dedication

Thank you for the blessings, inspiration, and support from:

Family:

Dear husband and friend: Raffaello Stefanini

Wonderful daughters: Vanessa Hart Margolis and Clelia Hart Stefanini

Father and consultant role model: Allan Joseph Schultz

Professional Colleagues:

Kajsa Brymdyr, Karin Cadwell, Cathy Watson Genna, Kay Hoover, Cindy Turner-Maffei

Healers and Practitioners:

Barbara d'Amato, Geraldine Hennessy Kelly, Elizabeth Ann Krimmel, Jacqueline Russell, Gandhi Nelson

Publishing Experts:

Nancy Zatzman, Kathy Kendall-Tackett, Janet Rourke

Musicians, Skaters, and Friends:

Christine Balfa, John Doyle, Lyn Hardy, Frances Kuber, Chuen-Gun Lee, Adam Rippon, Beverly Smith, Jay Ungar, Toni Williams, Carolyn Zimmerman

Every mother and baby I have served, for being the best teachers of all.

Table of Contents

Introduction

Breastfeeding rehabilitation and recovery can be achieved with the use of soft techniques and complementary and alternative therapies, including manual ones, where the therapist's hands are the tools. The International Board of Lactation Consultant Examiners (IBLCE) states that lactation consultants "have the duty to provide competent services for mothers and families by providing evidence-based information regarding complementary therapies during lactation and their impact on a mother's milk production and the effect on her child" (IBLCE, 2008).

There are challenges for lactation therapists that can't always be completely resolved by current lactation practices. What can be done when the baby has reflux or a torticollis? Or when both mother and baby are injured or in pain? Or when the mother can't relax enough to sleep? Or when she doesn't feel that the baby is hers, even while taking care of it? Or when weeks of pumping around the clock and bottle-feeding, and struggling to breastfeed erode her energy to the point of wanting to quit? These types of situations can benefit from the use of complementary and alternative medicine (CAM) in order to reach the goal of a thriving baby, a happy mother, an abundant milk supply, and easy breastfeeding.

CAM has been criticized in the past for lacking supportive evidence. Today, this is no longer true. Evidence-based healthcare is defined in the Cochrane Collaborative's online course, "Understanding Evidence-Based Healthcare: A Foundation for Action" as "the integration of best research evidence with clinical expertise and patient values" (Dickersin & Mayer, 2009). According to this definition, CAM is evidence-based healthcare.

This book contains wisdom and opinions gleaned from my history, education, and experience. Only a few of the many modalities classified as CAM will be discussed—ones with which I have had personal experience. It is a revelation to realize that at age 60, I have enough experience and education to have opinions and observations to share with practitioners, consultants, counselors, and therapists who work with breastfeeding dyads.

Complementary therapies and soft techniques, when used in conjunction with proven breastfeeding management or by a lactation therapist, do no harm and usually help the mother and baby to feel better, even if breastfeeding itself is lost. A mother who called for a consultation when she got home with her twins is an example of how a complementary therapy and a soft technique helped the mothering relationship, even when breastfeeding was not achieved. Her premature twins were released from the Intensive Care Nursery in a hospital the mother described as "breastmilk-friendly and not breastfeeding-friendly." The twins were five weeks old when they were discharged home. The mother called for a consultation with me shortly before her return to paid employment at six weeks postpartum. She chose craniosacral therapy out of all possible types of CAM because a friend had breastfeeding success after treatment. When our craniosacral therapy session was over, the babies were left skin-to-skin with their mother.

In the follow-up telephone call a few days later, the mother reported holding her babies skin-to-skin for five hours and discovering such intense joy that her mothering was transformed. She described feeling as if she had "taken her babies into her heart." She was never able to establish breastfeeding, probably because she had only one week between the consultation and her return to work, but she was able to relax and accept feeding her babies with her pumped milk and supplementing with formula. Subsequent follow-up found her sustaining skin-to-skin closeness and cuddling with her babies for the joy of it. She had become a mother in her own heart, instead of a caretaker.

Complementary and alternative therapies and soft techniques induce a parasympathetically driven state of calm, ease, and milk flow, like gentling a wild kitten, an angry child, or a fussy parent, a trait common to all types of CAM. A state of calm is healing—because stress is removed. There is release of tension because telling our unique story in our own time with a witness to our telling is therapeutic.

Complementary and Alternative Therapies in Lactation Therapy will give the reader an inside view of the modalities most familiar to me. I have become certified in some; in others, I have been the recipient. You, gentle reader, will have to seek further education to learn how to give these types of therapies. This book is NOT an instruction manual; it is an open door to the world of other ways of healing.

Complementary and Alternative Medicine (CAM)

In the 21st century, the Internet and global travel expanded public awareness of the many complementary and alternative medicines. Today, the delineation between 'conventional' and 'complementary' medicine is not as clear as it used to be.

In the last decades of the 20th century, complementary therapies were often viewed as those outside the common stream of conventional or standard (also called "Western" or "allopathic") medical practice. Standard Western medicine is a collection of healing techniques and services that one would find in a hospital, where laboratories, radiology departments, and other technologies are used to diagnose and treat illness and disease.

Physicians practice allopathic medicine. A physician is a graduate of a post-baccalaureate, accredited, four-year medical school, who has passed a licensing examination. After licensure, the physician is the authority for prescribed treatments, medications, and therapies. Other licensed practitioners with prescriptive authority in allopathic medicine are physician's assistants, nurse practitioners, nurse-midwives, and nurse-anesthetists.

The National Center for Complementary and Alternative Medicine (NCCAM), founded in 1998, is the U.S. government's agency for scientific research on medical and healthcare systems, practices, and products that are not part of conventional (also called 'allopathic') medicine. NCCAM has categorized complementary and alternative medicine into five groups: biologically based practices, manipulative/body-based practices, mind-body-based practices, whole medical systems, and energy medicine (Barnes, Bloom, & Nahin, 2008). Folk medicine practices, traditional healers, and religious and faith healing are not included.

Herbal medicines and special diets are biologically based practices. Chiropractic, osteopathy, craniosacral therapy, and massage are manipulative/body-based practices. Hypnosis and guided imagery are types of mind-body-based practices. Homeopathy and Chinese medicine are examples of whole medical systems. Reiki and therapeutic touch are examples of energetic medicine.

Barnes and colleagues and the American Cancer Society agree that complementary therapies are those to be used with conventional treatments, while alternative therapies are used in place of conventional treatment (Barnes et al., 2008). It is interesting to note that conventional medicine is sometimes considered "traditional," although it is only about 400 years old; whereas some of the modalities classified as CAM are thousands of years old.[1]

Conventional or allopathic medicine is defined as: "The treatment of disease by creating conditions which are opposite or hostile to the conditions resulting from the disease itself. Drugs and surgery are allopathic treatments. The term is sometimes used to refer to conventional Western medicine to contrast it with alternative therapies."[2] Another source defines conventional (allopathic) medicine as: "The traditional medicine of Western culture, which focuses on a specific disease or problem and treats it."[3]

As already stated, the definitions of "conventional," "alternative," and "complementary" are not as clear-cut as they were at the beginning of my career in healthcare in 1971. Sometimes common practices are defined by geography, as with herbal medicine that is a part of medical practice in Europe and China, and not in the U.S. Sometimes the boundaries are set by discipline; biofeedback is used in Physical Medicine and Rehabilitation, and yet is not part of allopathic medicine as a whole.[4] "The distinction between complementary and alternative medicine (CAM) and mainstream medicine has lessened as many practices have undergone rigorous research and have been increasingly integrated into mainstream care" (Kemper et al., 2008). Acupuncture was difficult to find in the States in the 1970s, but is now easily accessible. The Mayo Clinic recognizes the interest in and value of CAM and has published its *Guide to Alternative Medicine 2011*, which views the integration of CAM with conventional medicine as being the best of both worlds.

The debate about the effectiveness, validity, and reliability of complementary therapies lingers, with some organizations (Quackwatch.com being one) determined to prove ineffectiveness, and others (National Institutes of Health) using classic research methods for evaluation. It is important to remember that allopathic medicine lacks supporting evidence for some of its practices, such as the off-label use of medications or routine episiotomy. The use of randomized, clinically controlled trials is considered a gold standard to validate practice; yet, most routine obstetrical practices, accepted as standard by the legal system and by insurance companies, are

---

1   http://www.consultwebs.com/glossary/glossary-of-holistic-terms/a/
2   http://www.cancer.org/docroot/ETO/content/ETO_5_3x_Guidelines_For_Using_
     Complementary_and_Alternative_Methods.asp
3   http://www.yoga-free.com/content/glossary
4   http://en.wikipedia.org/wiki/Alternative_medicine

not supported by the Cochrane Collaborative and its universally acclaimed independent meta-analyses.

For some people, anything outside allopathic medicine is considered irrational, without value, and subject to variation outside the realm of predictability. There is a historical basis for the value of science in the allopathic model and the conflict between it and CAM.

A Brief History of Healing in the United States

For over 100 years, CAM has been viewed with skepticism and even disdain by the allopathic, conventional medical system. There are historical reasons for these attitudes.

In the 1830s, a popular health movement swept the U.S. This movement was the result of many societal trends: a reaction to forced medical professionalism when 13 states passed medical licensing laws, an emphasis on self-determination and self-sufficiency that has been called Jacksonian democracy, and a protest against the 'heroic' medical practices of the 18th century. The popular health movement was also a reaction to trained doctors, who, since the 1700s, had sought to elevate themselves above other healers. The middle and upper class people who could afford the higher fees chose to gain the prestige of being treated by a physician, although other practitioners didn't share this elevated view. Elizabeth Nihell, an 18th century midwife, lamented that the male physician "…used instruments unnecessarily to hasten the birth and save his own time, as well as to impress the family with his dexterity and justify charging a higher fee" (van Teijlingen, Porter, Lewis, & McCaffery, 2004).

Medical practices of the late 1700s to the end of the 1800s were aggressive: bloodletting, intestinal purging, vomiting, blistering, and sweating. Poisons were used for treatment, such as arsenic for the cure of syphilis. These treatments were the best that medicine could offer at the time. President Washington's death was probably hastened by these medical practices, as too much blood was taken from him.[5]

Medical training, even at the university level, was not formalized (medical courses ranged in length from two months to two years) and a high school diploma was not necessary for admission.

Another factor in the Popular Health Movement was a social class struggle, where working-class activists considered "King-craft, Priest-craft, Lawyer-

5   http://www.statemaster.com/encyclopedia/Natural-health

craft, and Doctor-craft" as evils of the time. The combination of social forces and energy resulted in an explosion of healing modalities, expressed in the popular saying, "Every man his own doctor." Women were also recognized as healers, deserving of education and respect. According to Ehrenreich and English (1973), "The peak of the Popular Health Movement coincided with the beginnings of an organized feminist movement, and the two were so closely linked that it's hard to tell where one began and the other left off."

Naturopathy, homeopathy, chiropractic, hydrotherapy, herbalism, Grahamism, eclectic medicine, and natural hygiene were popular during this time. Medical schools were open to African Americans, women, and working-class people. The goal of many medical schools was to graduate practitioners that would be readily affordable to the poor and middle class.

The regulars, as physicians of the 19th century were sometimes called, found themselves outnumbered and unpopular for several decades, while the populist health movement swept the nation. However, over time, the populist energy was diffused, as each branch of the health movement became isolated and combative with the other branches, giving the regular doctors a chance to regroup.

In 1848, a national association, the American Medical Association, was formed and began to attack lay and secular practitioners. One of its rallying points was the view that women could not be doctors or health practitioners because they were less capable than men, and that intellectual activity was injurious to their reproductive capacity. (As a nursing student in 1968, I was taught to stand up when a doctor entered the nurses' station, let him enter an elevator first, and surrender to him any patient's chart I was using–an artifact of this old attitude.)

Even though the regular doctors had formed a cohesive organization, they still had little dominance in the healing field until the occurrence of new developments in Europe. European research advanced the germ theory of disease. Antiseptic surgery and use of scientific method became integral parts of medical education, as the new scientific discoveries gave hope that disease could be conquered. A group of American doctors went to Europe to learn the new theories. In 1893, some of these German-trained doctors set up the first medical school in the U.S. based on the European model; this was the Johns Hopkins University in Baltimore, Maryland. Innovations developed at Hopkins put medical school out of reach for most of the public who could not afford four years of training after four years of college.

Around the same time as the medical profession was growing, U.S. industrial practices became a global force. Industrialists, looking to put their fortunes to good use, created foundations. Two are named after their founders, Rockefeller and Carnegie. One goal of these foundations was medical reform. Their power, political connections, and money were put behind the American Medical Association (AMA), the regulars, and medical schools. To qualify for foundation money, medical schools had to meet requirements that replicated the Hopkins model or go without funding. Around the same time, the AMA created a Council on Medical Education, whose goal was to modernize how medical students were taught. The Carnegie Foundation chose and paid for Abraham Flexner to make a tour of North America and evaluate 155 medical schools. At the time of Dr. Flexner's tour, medical schools varied greatly in their depth of education and training. Physicians ran some as moneymaking businesses; many were not part of a university. Dr. Flexner's report of his findings was published in 1910.

The Flexner Report (Flexner, 1910) still has an impact on medical training today. Besides standardizing admissions requirements (a high school diploma and a college education), medical education, and training, this powerful document had other consequences. Most of the medical schools for women, African-Americans, and the poor were closed because they didn't meet the new requirements and because there was an occult bias against them. Because the number of medical schools in the U.S. went from 160 in 1904 to 85 in 1920, the number of graduate doctors decreased. This enabled the doctors that were practicing to charge more money. In the 1950s, doctors were one of the wealthier social groups. When I graduated college with a BSN in 1972, many medical students that I knew spoke openly about their dreams of a wealthy life after starting a practice.

Another consequence of the Flexner Report was that all forms of healing that did not follow the biomedical model were considered quackery and bogus practice. Medical schools offering courses in populist medical disciplines had to stop or lose their accreditation. (Hahnemann Hospital, founded in 1885 in Philadelphia, was originally a homeopathic institution.) The regular physicians, heretofore just another group of practitioners, had gained power and prestige, and were now able to discredit all other disciplines, including midwifery. The regulars had become medical professionals, members of an elite group in a world where all other forms of healing science had been eliminated or subdued.[6]

Once medical doctors took control, birth moved from home to hospitals, as student doctors needed a population for practice, and it was more efficient

_____

6   http://en.wikipedia.org/wiki/Flexner_Report

to have many women in one place than to have one doctor traveling from home to home. The increase in hospital birth was concomitant with a drop in breastfeeding rates.

I was told by an assistant director of nursing at Osteopathic Hospital in Philadelphia (long-closed) that resident obstetricians had to practice techniques in order to be competent once they left training, even if women didn't need the intervention. She told me this to help me understand why resident obstetricians were doing unnecessary things to laboring women, like using a vacuum extractor on the baby during a precipitous labor.

Attitudes generated by the Flexner Report persist today in states that prosecute midwives for attending normal births, in the minds of insurance companies and governmental programs that refuse to pay for births in birth centers, and in a medical skepticism of complementary and alternative therapies. This attitude was manifested in the 1957 Article 3 of the AMA Principles of Medical Ethics, "A physician should practice a method of healing founded on a scientific basis, and he should not voluntarily professionally associate with anyone who violates this principle" (AMA, 1957).

In 1980, the AMA revised its code of Medical Ethics to include respecting "the rights of other healthcare professionals" and to "use the talents of other healthcare professionals when indicated" (AMA, 1980).

More History and Philosophy

Evidence from research and scientific process is a component of evidence-based healthcare, along with practitioner experience and client values (Sackett, 1997). In my baccalaureate nursing education, I was taught to value research studies and scientific thought, and to discard emotion and intuition as being "unscientific," unreliable sources of information. My undergraduate degree (1972) is a Bachelor of Science degree, nursing being a scientifically based discipline, developed to carry out orders issued by physicians in the dominant, allopathic system.

Evidence has been valued over emotion and intuition, beginning in the 17th century, when the concept of soul was considered to be separate from the physical world. Philosophers and scientists in the 1600s debated about the nature, importance, and relationship of the soul and the body, while new sciences emerged that were based on experimentation and measurement (Henry, 1987). Protestants of the 16th century, like Descartes, valued the new explorations of the physical world, which lead to the evolution of a dualistic theology, whereby the soul and the body were considered to be separate entities. The body functions and material world would be studied via the new sciences; the functions of the soul were left to the clergy. This split between mind and body is called dualism.

A simplistic view of dualism is that things are either matter (manifest in the physical world) or mind and spirit. Matter and physical form are studied with the tools of science; mind and spirit are explored in other ways. There is little overlap (Brennan, 1993). The essence of Descartes' philosophy can be distilled into a mechanistic view: the whole is the sum of all its parts. If one part isn't working, then that part must be fixed for the whole to function.

Processed food reflects a mechanistic view of nutrients. Processed food is a collection of nutrient parts. Consider chicken fingers, a cheap and popular food made from a paste of ground up chicken parts extruded into standard-sized shapes and deep-fried. No chicken has fingers, yet today, children are learning otherwise. In a lecture by popular author Michael Pollan,[7] he speaks about food losing its dynamism and becoming instead a collection of manufactured nutrients that he calls "edible, food-like substances."

The view of something as merely a collection of parts is also called reductionist. A recent example of reductionist education was described in a New York Times interview with T. Colin Campbell, PhD, co-author of the book *The China Study* (Parker-Pope, 2011). Dr. Campbell spoke about his early education in nutrition, where he studied one nutrient at a time, out of context, "a reductionist, narrowly-focused way." He then speaks of learning from his work in the Philippines and in China that it is most important to think about how things work together.

The formula industry practices reductionist thinking in their constant drive to improve human milk substitutes, i.e., infant formula. When a new component of human milk is identified, the formula industry manufactures it in a laboratory and adds it to their product. This "new, improved" formula is then marketed to the public. However, as formula has to be a dead, sterile substance, so it can sit on a shelf for months without spoiling, it can never come close to living, dynamic human milk.

Giving drugs to suppress symptoms is another illustration of a mechanistic view of the body. Hiding symptoms is like a driver using earplugs to mask the sound of a flapping flat tire. One can get away with the hiding or masking for a while, but eventually there is illness to the person or damage

---

7   http://www.youtube.com/watch?v=OjutojvbsTg&feature=channel

to the structure of the car. Many medicines prescribed today do not cure any illness; they merely make a symptom go away. The statin drugs do not cure or modify what is going on in a person's body that deranges healthy metabolism. One is supposed to take statins for the rest of one's life to deal with an unhealthy lipid profile and have liver function tests every three months to monitor for side effects. Allopaths rarely perform any in-depth assessment of a person's whole self (body, mind, and soul) to determine the underlying reason for the high cholesterol level.

The split between soul and body was a mainstream attitude until the 1960s. Then, new experiences and inner reality caught the public's attention. Global travelers discovered other sources of wisdom and healing practices in Asia and India and brought them home. When President Nixon established relations with China, he also opened the door to cross-cultural communication in medicine and philosophy, along with politics and economics. New ideas were brought to public attention (in part through the activities of musicians and celebrities), thus widening people's perspectives to include Chinese medicine, ayurveda, transcendental meditation, osteopathy, chiropractic, homeopathy, and massage. Some of the Beatles talked about transcendental meditation and Primal Therapy®, increasing public awareness through their own explorations. Research into the different functions of right and left-brains expanded the acceptance of new ideas, building on a concept developed earlier in the 20th century, namely that emotions can create disease.

Dr. Walter Cannon in the 1920s and Dr. Hans Selye in the 1950s both researched and published about links between emotions and disease. Dr. Cannon developed the concept of "flight or fight" to express the function of the sympathetic nervous system as it responded to psychological or physical threats by raising blood pressure and heart rate, and increasing the acuity of hearing and vision.

Dr. Selye's work carried studies of nervous system physiology further and stated that everybody responds to stress in the same way; this universal response is called the General Adaptation Syndrome. Other systems respond to stress along with the nervous system; the endocrine system releases different hormones, the digestive system reduces its activity, and immune and restorative functions are inhibited. Dr. Selye suggested that people under chronic stress would get sick more often, as their adaptation to stress kept their body systems functioning in arousal or sympathetic mode, with resultant ulcers and infections. Chronic stress impedes growth and healing (Richmond, 2010). Modern science was beginning to recognize a link between the mind and the body, although it took a few decades for the concepts to become familiar to the public.

The renaissance of interest and exploration into the power of the mind both led to and grew out of the consciousness-raising movements of the late 1950s, the 1960s, and the 1970s, where there was a revival of some of the populist health movements from a century earlier. A general interest in personal responsibility for one's health, a belief in one's personal power, and a zest for social activism fueled this revival. Self-help groups became popular during this era. Students demonstrated against the Vietnam war and for change in educational systems. Betty Friedan published *The Feminine Mystique* in 1963 that inspired women to question the status quo and break away from societal norms to explore new roles. The Boston Women's Health Collective printed the first edition of *Our Bodies, Our Selves*, written by women for women about women's health issues. This popular book contained practical information about abortion, contraception, sexually transmitted diseases, pregnancy, birth, and breastfeeding in a style that was easily understood. No longer did women have to rely on allopathic practitioners for all the information.

Childbirth education associations formed as a reaction to the drugged, numbed births of the 20s, 30s, and 50s; the earliest were the International Childbirth Education Association and ASPO/Lamaze in 1960. Mother-to-mother support for breastfeeding spread across the world, starting with seven mothers meeting in a park in Chicago, Illinois, in 1956; this meeting was the foundation for La Leche League. What all of these activities had in common was a tremendous interest in self-help and grassroots organization. During those years, women could spend 40 or more hours a week doing volunteer work, and did so. I remember those times as full of joy, excitement, and intense passion.

After 30 years of an increase in health awareness and education, and an interest in alternative and complementary therapies, the national government responded. In 1998, the National Center for Complementary and Alternative Medicine was founded by the Federal Government, an official and formal recognition of interest in therapies and healing modalities outside allopathy. The NCCAM has a budget of nearly $130 million dollars a year and has 65 full-time employees. It is "the lead agency for scientific research on the diverse medical and healthcare systems, practices, and products that are not generally considered part of conventional medicine."[8]

The Nixon administration believed that profit should be part of healthcare; this was manifested in the creation of the health maintenance organization and diagnosis-related groups. For the first time in U.S. history, business concepts were applied to healthcare. Instead of medical practitioners deciding how much care was necessary for any medical condition, business

8   http://nccam.nih.gov/about/

administrators were making those decisions based on efficiency and cost savings. The attitudes, beliefs, ideas, and practices that were an outgrowth of the profit motive worked against the populist health movement, as government agencies took control, regulating in favor of corporations and standard practices. Today, politics and profit reign. Several examples of this relevant to breastfeeding are the regulations against the use of domperidone as a galactagogue, and the lack of reimbursement by most insurance plans for lactation therapy.

Today, healthcare is standardized to ensure that everyone receives the same care, so the individual practitioner can be protected from legal action. Allopathy is often practiced in a factory model, aiming for mass production at the lowest expense, where practitioners may see 30 to 60 clients in a clinic workday, and where Philadelphia hospitals close their maternity units because of insufficient remuneration by government agencies and by insurance companies. As an increasing percentage of clients are uninsured or uninsurable, the financial impact of birth is increased to tax payers. In the early 1990s, I remember reading a Philadelphia newspaper reporting on the closing of a hospital's maternity unit that quoted a manager as saying that "birth is non-productive." From a corporate viewpoint, birth, the process of producing our young, is considered valueless because it doesn't generate income.

At the beginning of the 1900s, the factory approach, and the assembly line, were considered to be modern and efficient, and were enthusiastically applied to schools and hospitals. In the 21st century, there is a strong trend towards improving the efficiency of hospitals by turning them into 'focused factories' (Leung, 2000), as "one solution to our current efficiency and productivity crisis."

While the factory approach is efficient when building cars, it is not effective or pleasant when applied to the health of the living. The focus of the factory is the product. When a dynamic, physiologic process, like labor, is manipulated according to a factory model (Kato, Nagata, Furuya, Seki, & Makimura, 1994), one can understand another reason for a national cesarean section rate of 32.3% in 2008.

Another consequence of the mechanistic viewpoint is the fragmentation of healthcare in the U.S. Breastfeeding professionals and pediatricians both lament the lack of communication between obstetricians and pediatricians. The obstetricians get the baby out; the pediatricians are left to pick up the pieces if the baby is premature or injured as a result of obstetrical practices. In my work in public health, I hear each part of the healthcare system complain about the other parts. I've heard pediatricians complain about obstetricians, hospital practitioners complain about community providers, community providers complain about hospital staff, nurses complain about physicians, physicians complain about nurses, and providers complain about clients. There is no big picture, only fragments that blame other fragments for problems. Creating a cohesive system is one of the major challenges in healthcare in the U.S. of the 21st century.

The drive to profit increases fragmentation. When my last baby was intubated after delivery due to a 43+ week gestation, variable decelerations in labor, and thick meconium at birth, each segment of the pediatric procedure had its own charge and billing code: one charge to put the tube down her throat, another to look through the tube, and a third charge to remove it.

In a factory, every worker on the assembly line has one unique job that is performed all day long on the assembly line. This takes less time and results in more automobiles manufactured than if one person built the whole automobile. The aim of the manufacturing process is speed; consequently, efficiency and profit become highly valued. The scientific view assumes that systems follow predefined rules to achieve their objectives, which are externally determined. Newton argued in the *General Scholium* that "the universe was created with all its governing laws, so it can function like clockwork without the day to day interference of the creator spirit" (Saraswat, 1998). [9]

The downside of the factory approach, with its scientific viewpoint and its emphasis on efficiency and productivity, is that it ignores or discounts the importance of time, safety, feelings, and warmth for the physiologic responses that are necessary for birth, breastfeeding, and relationship.

Birth is more than the sum of a number of contractions, lasting however long they should at each stage, with how long it takes to push the baby out. A healthy baby is more than the sum of its feeds, pees, poops, and weight gain. The only factory recognition of emotion is the consideration of bonding between mother and baby after delivery; dyads are given one hour to fall in love in the delivery room. This fluid, varying, and sensitive process of falling in love is given a precise timed interval before the mother and baby are separated from each other and taken to different processing and recovery areas.

Skepticism of the energetic world, the world of the soul and feelings, and all the modalities related to work in its arena, has been endemic and today is fortunately shrinking. It is easy to count and measure and weigh. It is easy to treat everyone with a similar set of symptoms in the same way. It is easy to hold a measure of gold in our hands and weigh it, and difficult

9   http://www.rosenthal.hs.columbia.edu/MD_Courses.html

to evaluate the movement of a chakra. Yet, without all of ourselves—mind, body, and soul together, we cannot heal completely or function at our highest level of health.

Comparatively new disciplines, like psychology (about 100 years old) and psychoneuroimmunology (a term coined in 1964), make the mind-body connection the focus of clinical practice. Increasing numbers of medical and nursing schools are offering courses and electives about CAM. This is a new and welcomed development over the 35 years of my professional career.[10]

Energy Medicine

Energy medicine is the practice of medicine that evaluates and uses the flow of energy. In this paradigm, the physical body is seen as an organ of the energetic one, and what happens in the energetic field transmits to the physical field. Some practitioners, like Barbara Brennan, PhD, a former NASA scientist and expert in atmospheric physics, find that practicing with the energetic body in view first will help the physical body, as the energetic body is the matrix for the physical body template.

Energy is difficult to define. We learn in high school that it is the ability to do work. It has also been defined as the fundamental source that animates living things. One reference[11] states, "Energetic Medicine or Energy Medicine is the practice of medicine using energy or the flow of energy as a medium for healing. It is based on the biophysics of the body, whereas traditional medicine is, for the most part, based on biochemistry through the use of pharmaceuticals."

Neuroanatomist Jill Taylor, PhD, writes, "Although most of us are rarely aware of it, our sensory receptors are designed to detect information at the energy level. Because everything around us—the air we breathe, even the materials we use to build with—is composed of spinning and vibrating atomic particles, you and I are literally swimming in a turbulent sea of electromagnetic fields" (Taylor, 2006). In other words, we are all creatures with energy fields and energetic perceptions.

Feelings are a type of energy. Most of us have a special being in our lives. The way we feel about that person or pet or plant cannot be bottled or measured, yet is essential to our life's health and comfort. Practitioners do not yet routinely ask pregnant women if they are happy. Not everyone asks

---

10   http://www.energetic-medicine.net/energy-medicine.html
11   http://www.cvtoolbox.com/downloads/PhysEx/Combined_Templ.pdf

the new mother if she is having fun with her baby. Yet happiness and fun tell more about health than the mother's heart beating regularly within the accepted range of 60 to 80 beats per minute.

A challenge for some energetic modalities categorized as CAM is that their measure is often taken by the rules that govern the physical world; sometimes the current methods of research conclude that the therapy is ineffective. An example of this is craniosacral therapy, which has its own chapter.

Energetic modalities often involve a quality of spontaneity and intention that is not easily quantifiable. Imagine the question, "How much love does a baby need?" "Oh, at least 33 units a day." Such an answer is meaningless. We all know that love is essential to a hale and hearty life, but can it be measured?

Everyone has experience with the energetic world. Imagine being early for an event. Being the first to enter the empty room, you look around the room, and then select the seat that feels right. That "feeling right" is not measurable and cannot be randomized in a double-blind study, yet it is as real and important to one's comfort, learning, and participation as light, noise, and temperature levels.

An experiment to appreciate the power of energy is to stand facing the back wall of a crowded elevator and pay attention to internal sensations. No one says anything. It is a free country and we can stand in an elevator any way we choose. Yet the sense of facing the wrong way is strong and may motivate us to turn around.

Life-force energy is called Chi or Qi or Prana or Spirit, depending on the framework, and is not always formally evaluated in Western medicine. For example, a current template for assessment of heart function does not include feelings, energy, beliefs, or attitudes that have a bearing on the patient's condition.[12]

One general difference between Western and Eastern medicine has been in their study of the human body. Western medicine has been based on the study of dead things, things that can be dissected, looked at under a microscope, or broken into components to be analyzed in a laboratory. Eastern medicine has been based on the study of live creatures, dynamic and moving. Some allopathic practitioners are skeptical of craniosacral therapy because they learned in their anatomy classes in medical school that bone does not move. Healthcare professional students study dead bone or plastic models. Dead bone cannot move; live bone does.

12   http://www.simmsmanncenter.ucla.edu/

Times are changing. New technologies are blurring the boundaries between Eastern and Western medical paradigms. The work of Dr. Donna (Ramsey) Geddes and her colleagues at the University of Western Australia is a lovely, modern example. The common view of internal breast anatomy comes from Dr. Astley Cooper's drawings based on cadaver dissection done in the 1840s. In the 21st century, Australian researchers used real-time ultrasound to look inside the breast to see what happened during a breastfeed and during milk ejection (Ramsey, Kent, Hartmann, & Hartmann, 2005; Geddes, 2009). Ultrasound is now used to measure and evaluate breast structures (Gooding, Finlay, Shipley, Halliwell, & Duck, 2010), a heretofore unimaginable technology.

Breastfeeding professionals can now see the reason for the first minute latch-on pain described by Lawrence (1994) and Lee (1997). The intensity and sudden onset of this transient and often painful sensation comes from milk ducts suddenly expanding to five times their diameter in a matter of seconds after the baby has started to suckle; ultrasound imaging has made Dr. Cooper's drawings obsolete.

The Current State of CAM

A new trend in medicine is called 'integrative therapy' and blends CAM and allopathic medicine. Researchers at the Simms/Mann-ULCLA Center for Integrative Oncology are finding that patients fighting cancer want both CAM and conventional treatments. CAM is useful in attaining spiritual and psychological fulfillment and relieving side effects and symptoms, while the conventional chemotherapy and radiation therapies do their work.[13]

UCLA and the University of Arizona are examples of modern universities that have a large program of integrative medicine. At UCLA, it is called the ULCA Collaborative Centers for Integrative Medicine. Within the collaboration is the Center for East-West Medicine, the Center for Human Nutrition, the Cousins Center for Psychoneuroimmunology, the Mindful Awareness Research Center, the Center for Neurovisceral Sciences and Women's Health, the Pediatric Pain Program at Mattel Children's Hospital UCLA, and the Stiles Program for Integrative Oncology. At the University of Arizona, the CAM training and research program is targeted to pre- and post-doctoral students. The concept of collaboration and cooperation between different healing modalities is the wave of the future.

The UCLA program was the first hit in a Google search for the topic, "combining eastern and western medicine;" 209,000 total sites were listed.

13   http://nccam.nih.gov/health/financial/

Some are university programs (such as UCLA) and others are private practitioners who offer a range of skills. In the 21st century, blending elements of standard lactation management (aides and devices, physical and education strategies for latch-on and positioning, drugs and galactagogues) with CAM is right in style.

The Economics of CAM

CAM is big business. In the article "Use of unconventional therapies by individuals with multiple sclerosis" (Nayak, Matheis, Schoenberger, & Shiflett, 2003), the authors state, "The most common reason for using CAM was the desire to use holistic healthcare (i.e., treatments that recognized the interrelatedness of mind, body, and spirit) and dissatisfaction with conventional medicine." The authors speculate that over half of the people with MS are using CAM; the most common modalities used are herbal remedies, manipulation, massage, and acupuncture. The state of medicine is in flux about CAM now, in part because the public is spending so much money on it that conventional medicine is both curious and seeking to divert the cash flow into its own coffers.

Reimbursement implies recognition by the mainstream insurance industry. The National Center for Complementary and Alternative Medicine says, "Not all health insurance plans offer CAM coverage, however. When they do, the coverage varies by state and is often limited. Examples of CAM therapies that are sometimes covered by insurance are chiropractic, acupuncture, massage therapy, biofeedback, and naturopathy. Consumers' interest in CAM coverage is prompting more insurance companies and managed care organizations to consider offering this coverage as an option."[14]

"Americans spent $33.9 billion out-of-pocket on complementary and alternative medicine (CAM) over the previous 12 months" according to a 2007 government survey (Nahin, Barnes, Stussman, & Bloom, 2009). Barnes and colleagues (2008) state that one in four adults, and one in nine children had used CAM in the 12 months prior to being surveyed.

Why People Seek CAM

One reason people choose CAM is that practitioners offer something that is in scant supply in standard medical practice: time. A typical doctor-patient encounter takes 18.3 to 21.5 minutes (Mechanic, McAlpine, & Rosenthal, 2001). A visit with a complementary practitioner can take between one

14   www.cochrane.org/reviews

and three hours. Time to tell the whole story uncovers clues and patterns a practitioner can use to provide individualized care. Telling one's story is another part of healing. Most of us are familiar with the relief that comes from telling the story of a significant event to interested listeners. This story telling is part of the benefit of mother-to-mother and of self-help support groups, where a person is free to speak until they are finished, and where there is no pressure to tell the story in a set time-period.

In a study of midwives in New Zealand and Canada, the reasons for the use of CAM by midwives were grouped into four categories: resistance, efficacy, women's (or client's) choice, and keeping birth normal. Midwives want to avoid medical intervention and use natural remedies because the remedies are gentle and effective, with fewer side effects than allopathic ones. Sometimes it is the client who chooses CAM, and the midwives honor that choice, as it encourages the client to take more control and responsibility in their own care (Harding & Foureur, 2009).

The Cochrane Collaboration has 83 published reviews of CAM,[15] covering a range of clinical situations. Some CAM is effective (e.g., acupuncture and hypnosis in managing the pain of labor and avocado soybean unsaponifiables for treating osteoarthritis), some need further research to establish efficacy, and some (such as herbal medicine for the treatment of HIV and AIDS) have thus far proved to be ineffective. Most of the CAM reviews published find merit in further study, as preliminary results are intriguing.

The Value of CAM in Lactation Practice

Complementary therapies, when used in conjunction with proven breastfeeding management, do no harm and may help the mother and baby feel better with each other, even if breastfeeding is lost. Case histories to illustrate will be presented in subsequent chapters.

As breastfeeding therapists are working with two people (mother and baby) within the context of their history, family, culture, and experience, time is an essential quality of the therapeutic relationship. Unlike a mother, a baby cannot be rushed or pressured into cooperating. Different behaviors emerge when the environment permits the situation to unfold without the pressure of having to finish the visit by a pre-determined hour.

A major hormone that influences milk flow and release via the milk ejection reflex (or "letdown") requires a level of maternal relaxation for its release,

---

15 http://www.healthgrades.com/media/dms/pdf/PatientSafetyInAmericanHospitalsStudy2006. pdf

particularly at the beginning of lactation. Many complementary therapies induce a state of relaxation. Nearly 100 years ago, Hans Selye found that a stressful situation does not promote healing or tissue repair. A newer study connects anger with delayed wound healing (Gouin, Kiecolt-Glaser, Malarkey, & Glaser, 2008). CAM often creates a safe environment and gives time for the dyad to relax together.

Complementary therapies are useful, and when used consciously and carefully, make the client happy and cause no harm. Views of health and healing vary among people. There is more than one approach to a problem. Some people enjoy the control they have over their own care, as with homeopathy, where a person can learn about self-treatment, purchase remedies at low cost, and treat common conditions in family members.

Ensuring Safety

Practitioner safety, talent, and reliability are concerns in any healing work. There are regular news reports on the side effects of prescription medications or of poor hospital and medical practices that cause injury or death. In 2000, Dr. Barbara Starfield (2000) published an article stating that medical errors are a leading cause of death in the United States.

Dr. Starfield's report included some frightening statistics: there were 2,000 deaths per year from unnecessary surgery; 7,000 deaths per year from medication errors in hospitals; 20,000 deaths per year from other errors in hospitals; 80,000 deaths per year from infections in hospitals; 106,000 deaths per year from non-error, adverse effects of medications. In the U.S., 225,000 deaths per year are from iatrogenic causes, the Number Three killer. In April 2006, the Third Annual Patient Safety in American Hospital study stated that medical errors are an increasing cause of patient injury and death, and not all states have mandatory reporting of adverse events.

Iatrogenic means adverse effects or complications caused by medical treatments, whether it is from misdiagnosis, interference with natural process, or reactions from prescribed medications. Currently 42% of singleton preterm births in the U.S. are iatrogenic in origin, the result of obstetrical intervention (MacDorman, Declercq, & Zhang, 2010). Allopathy has its weaknesses, just as CAM does.

"Caveat emptor" (Let the buyer beware) is an old saying, and is still true. One must pay attention, and be conscious and involved with one's therapy. If there is no improvement in breastfeeding after three treatments, consider a different modality or a different practitioner. Using a practitioner recommended by trusted sources is an excellent way to ensure safety; word of mouth is the best marketing.

Beware of the easy fix, where instant results are promised after a short time, and often with a significant expense. If long travel is necessary to meet with a practitioner, have enough conversation with that practitioner to feel respected, heard, and valued before investing in the journey. There should be enough positive reports from others that the long journey is justified.

Ideally, all practitioners are sensible about their responsibilities to the public—to do no harm, to provide the best and safest care, and to provide follow-up. Speaking truth, in language the client understands, and taking the time to assess the client's understanding are part of safety and professional accountability.

It is not possible to do more in this book than present a thumbnail sketch of the history behind the attitudes and interactions between allopathy and CAM. My intention is to engage the reader and to encourage exploration, tolerance, and integration of some of the concepts or practices. One does not have to believe in anything for it to work. If that were true, homeopathic remedies would be useless for babies and animals who are unable to believe in anything. And, if truth be told, the complete reasons that many modern medical practices work cannot be identified either. Welsh poet Dylan Thomas made a comment in *A Child's Christmas in Wales* about a gift book that "told everything about the wasp but why." Think of Shakespeare who said, "There are more things in Heaven and Earth, Horatio, than are dreamt of in your philosophy" (Hamlet, Act I, scene V).

When the usual strategies of pumping, latch assistance, strategies to modify milk production, and positioning guidance are not enough to resolve the breastfeeding challenge in a few weeks, consider the use of CAM. Table 1 provides an overview of some CAM in breastfeeding management.

Table 1. Overview of Some CAM in Breastfeeding Management

Modality	Basic education	Certified, licensed or lay practitioner	Enough by itself for breastfeeding rehabilitation. (All may be useful in conjunction with standard lactation management.)
Feng Shui	Self-education	Certified or Lay	No
Homeopathy	Formal study	Certified or Licensed	Possibly
Massage	Formal study	Certified, Licensed or Lay	Probably not
Craniosacral Therapy	Formal study	Certified	Possibly
Lymphatic Drainage Therapy	Formal study	Certified	Possibly
Acupuncture	Formal study	Licensed	Possibly
Chiropractic	Formal study	Licensed	Possibly
Osteopathy	Formal study	Licensed	Possibly

Creating the Healing Environment

Humans seek safety zones, geographical spaces where they feel safe enough to sleep, to heal, and recover, and to have intimate activity; places where they can be vulnerable to potential injury while feeling protected. To let our guard down, we choose an area that has only a few trusted people in it, so we can block out the outer world and tune in to our inner one.

Particular human activities take place in specialized environments. A stadium is a high-energy environment, full of noise, lights, action, smells, and excitement. The environment in a place of worship is different from a stadium, which is different from a classroom. Operating rooms are sterile, tiled for easy cleaning, and kept cool to increase the comfort for heavily garbed staff. The Newborn Individualized Developmental Care and Assessment Program (NIDCAP) provides guidance for making an intensive care nursery calm and restful for a premature infant to support its growth and development. We feel and behave differently, depending on our environment. Creating an environment where the dyad feels safe and comfortable, and where the practitioner gives complete attention, sets the stage for the optimal therapeutic relationship.

There are many ways to create healing environments. One way is to put mother and baby skin-to-skin with each other in a safe place and leave them alone. Skin-to-skin is the most basic and simple environment for the baby. This is a reliable strategy, a splendid way to assess the mother-infant relationship and to facilitate breastfeeding. Skin-to-skin is such a mighty topic that it has its own chapter.

Some practitioners designate a special room for healing work, and fill this room with thoughtfully chosen items and furnishings to create an environment that feels right. Qualities of light, color, sound, temperature, texture, placement of furnishings, and smell can transform a room into a sanctuary. A sanctuary is a sacred place, a place of refuge, a place where those within are protected.

When using a special room is not possible, as in the hospital, the practitioner can create a sense of sanctuary in a busy postpartum unit by closing the door to the mother's room, dimming the lights, drawing the curtain around her bed to protect her privacy (should the door be opened without warning), and turning off the television. An internal, personal sanctuary can be as easy as three deep and full consecutive breaths between one patient's room and another's, or mentally counting to ten before speaking (Kundtz, 1998).

Another way to create a healing environment is to use principles from Feng Shui, the science of environment.

Feng Shui

The Chinese science known as Feng Shui speaks directly to safe environment and energy flow. Its original concepts were derived from Chinese astronomy. The first mentions of placement of doors for optimal energy flow were in 4000 BC.

The goal of feng shui is to maximize the flow of good energy in any constructed space, such as cities, homes, and offices, so businesses flourish and the internal atmosphere is peaceful. There are many styles and forms of feng shui, many certified consultants for hire, and many books, articles, and Internet sites. As with other energetic practices, feng shui is revered by those who have had positive experiences with it and scorned by critics for being nonsense.

In March, 2010, the Disney Corporation modified the entrance to its theme park in Hong Kong after consultation with a feng shui master. The front gates were originally designed "to be in a straight line parallel to the octagonal square in front of them." The new design has the front gates "form(ing) an angle of 12 degrees to ensure prosperity." The main walkway had its course changed from the original straight path to an angled one to prevent positive energy from flowing into the sea. One hotel on the site had its location shift to receive positive energy; another hotel integrated motifs of feng shui elements (metal, water, fire, earth, and wood) for the same purpose. The design changes were made to honor local traditions, as a company from outside the culture (in this case, Disney) needs local approval to attract business. Whether the increased business is the consequence of Feng Shui, or the welcoming political and social climate engendered by Disney in honoring local customs, doesn't matter (Holson, 2005).

Landscape architects and ecologists, environmental scientists, and geographers all make use of principles of Feng Shui. Experts can be hired, but there is enough published on the Internet about Feng Shui that anyone can learn enough to create a lovely, healing space.

In an office, the goal is for money to flow in, so sit facing the door instead of with your back to it. Sitting in the corner farthest from the entrance gives you an "in charge" position; facing the entrance feels safer than having people come into the room from behind you.

I sometimes work in a cubicle, where it is not possible to rearrange the furniture. As a result, my chair has its back to the cubicle entrance, and sudden visitors have startled me. They are startled in turn by my shocked reaction. The solution came from an energy worker, who advised putting a red scarf on the back of my office chair. The energy of the color is protective, and it works. While I am surprised when someone suddenly enters, I no longer fall off my chair.

My Sanctuary

In the following picture, the massage table is usually along the right wall and is brought out into the middle of the floor only when being used. I chose everything in the room deliberately. It is very comfortable. Babies are fascinated by the contrast of the white ceiling with its dark beams. There is a bathroom nearby, and a entrance separate from the rest of the house. The windows and door face the woods. In spring, summer, and fall, the view is spectacular. Sun always comes in the room; prisms hanging in the windows cast dancing rainbows.

The picture below was taken in summer; all the plants are outside.

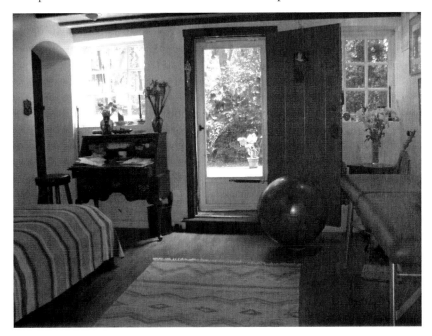

Figure 1. My sanctuary.

There is a big rocking chair out of view in this picture. When the weather is right, I've moved the chair outside to the patio, and worked with a dyad outside. Privacy is maintained.

My family is either away or knows to stay away when I have a client. My office is a place where I write, think, do yoga, practice music, and sometimes sleep when my husband snores too loudly. I use the physio-ball of the Planet Earth to sit on when I am working at the massage table. There are six places (including a dining room chair and pillows on the floor) where a mother can choose to sit.

Hospitals–The Opposite Of Sanctuaries

Imagine being a new mother, trying to connect with your baby in the intimate act of breastfeeding. Are you in a safe, private, and calm space? Or are you in a depersonalized room, where strangers come in and out all day long, and at least once an hour at night?

Birth and breastfeeding initiation often occurs in an atmosphere similar to that of the lobby of a busy train station. The mother keeps herself guarded because strangers are looking at and touching her sex organs and discussing her breasts. Her attendants are mostly strangers, who are conscious of doing everything according to policy to guard themselves against lawsuits, and who have long checklists of tasks that must be performed prior to discharge. Tasks not completed are left for the next shift. There is a subtle pressure for nursing staff to complete as many tasks as possible so the next shift will have less to do, thus maintaining a comfortable relationship with other staff members. As most women are only in the hospital for 48 hours and most nurses have more patients than can be handled in a relaxed manner, the atmosphere can be less than serene.

How can the new mother be expected to use her bared breasts when the door can open at any moment and a stranger come in? Dr. Barbara Morrison calculated that a new mother is interrupted an average number of 54 times in 12 hours in a tertiary urban hospital, and that half of her time alone with her infant is for nine minutes or less. Most of the interruptions are medical and nursing staff, next are dietary and housekeeping personnel, and visitors are third (Morrison, Ludington-Hoe, & Anderson, 2006).

How safe would a person need to feel to make love? That's how safe and relaxed a brand new mother needs to feel before she can open up to her baby and let go of her milk. In addition to feeling safe, each mother needs to go at her own pace. Some experienced mothers will feel safe within a matter of hours; primiparas can take weeks. If the mother is in pain or is injured, it may take her longer to relax. Safety and relaxation are inter-twined.

Many birthing places, save for home and freestanding birth centers, lack a feeling of safety. Birth centers on the hospital campus lead to unjustifiably high rates of transfers. Birth centers in hospitals can have environments that start out feeling safe, but can quickly turn judgmental. In one local birth center where I worked, one mother in five was transferred to the hospital because they "needed Pitocin,™" according to one midwife. Women find it difficult to relax into labor when they are told they must deliver in a particular amount of time to avoid intervention. Laboring women can be told that if they don't push the baby out in two or three hours, they will have a cesarean section. What sort of environment does the intention behind that statement create?

Some women benefit from absolute control over who enters their personal space. In one memorable case, intuition led me to leave my office door open, with a note on the floor saying "Welcome. Gone for a short walk. Back soon. Come in." This enabled the client to take possession of the space in any way she chose. This intuition arose after hearing her story when she called to make an appointment. Adrienne spoke of having three non-stress tests a week for 20 weeks to monitor a suspected two-vessel cord, of being told by different physicians that there were terrible things wrong with her baby, and of being reminded at every visit that she couldn't grow a healthy baby. She spent the last half of her pregnancy having her confidence steadily undermined. Leaving my office open gave her complete control over the environment, an opposite experience to what she had had, and one that laid the ground work for an atmosphere of safety.

When I returned from my walk, she'd settled on the sofa. She spoke about the arduous treatment she received during pregnancy. After 20 weeks of negative comments from her obstetricians and constant monitoring by machines, a miracle occurred–she had an "ecstatic" labor. She is the first and only woman in 35 years of my clinical practice to use that adjective to describe labor. She described a companion feeling of gleefulness, "See, my baby is fine!" She felt like she had "showed them," "them" being the healthcare staff that had doubted her and her baby for 20 weeks.

She wept while talking of still wanting to breastfeed six months after delivery, despite the induction and all the pain and loss of her dreams of easy mothering and breastfeeding. Her baby was given formula in the hospital against her stated and written wishes. She told me, "They didn't understand my anger. Nobody tried to help me breastfeed." She described herself as an extremely modest woman who "hates being naked and hates being open physically." She talked about feeling helpless and lost after the delivery. She told of missing the feeling of mothering her baby, even though he was in her arms and she did her best to act like a mother should.

She didn't feel safe to bare her breasts because she had to share her hospital room with a roommate.

Feeding him meant pumping and bottle-feeding her milk eight times a day for six months. How she was caring for her baby had no relation to the dreams she'd had while pregnant.

The woman that couldn't breastfeed in the hospital out of modesty bared her torso the instant I explained skin-to-skin care to her. She and her baby wrapped themselves around each other as she told their story, and the release of righteous emotions was witnessed and validated. I used craniosacral therapy techniques while she spoke, always staying in contact with her, imagining currents of energy moving through me into her. My intention was to soothe her core with my hands.

When the visit was over, three hours later, her husband was waiting to bring her home. I will always remember the lightness with which she danced out of my office, with her upturned face radiating joy and hope, as she told her husband all about it. The ultimate resolution of this case was a decision to abandon the struggle to breastfeed, to continue pumping and bottle-feeding, and to have as much fun and cuddling with her baby as possible. In other words, she chose to engage in joyful mothering of her precious baby.

Baby-Friendly™ practices, as described in the 10 Steps to Successful Breastfeeding, are guidelines for creating an environment that promotes breastfeeding. Unfortunately, out of about 3,000 maternity units in the U.S., as of February, 2011, only 105 are Baby-Friendly (Baby Friendly USA, 2011). In 2008, over 25% of breastfed babies received formula before two days of age (CDC, 2010a). In most hospitals in my neighborhood, mothers go home with their new baby and samples and coupons for formula are in the microfiber diaper bag they're given. Such an environment does not foster exclusive breastfeeding.

Creating Your Own Sanctuary

Think about your office. How does it make you feel to be there? How do your clients feel about it? How is the light in your workspace? There are two points of view about light. One is the view that you and your clients will be connected to the world when the light coming through windows changes with the seasons. The other view is that some people feel safest in a cave, where light is always dim and space is more contained. Which do you prefer?

Remember that the baby will often be looking up at the ceiling. Some ceiling or fluorescent lights can be so bright that the baby will keep its eyes closed and be reluctant to reach out.

How does your space smell? Do you and your clients enjoy its special odor? Smell is a sense that can be used in healing. Aromatherapy is the ancient science of using essential oils for healing via olfactory or tactile routes. Babies cried less and slept better when lavender-scented bath oil was added to their bathwater. The cortisol levels of mothers and babies were lower in the lavender-scented bath group than in the controls, who bathed in unscented water (Field, Field, et al., 2008). Friendly smells can be added with essential oils, candles, or incense.

Explore your space; imagine seeing it for the first time. Consider the placement of your desk and chair in relation to the door, the placement of plants, and the shape and color of your desk. Strive to balance the contrasts: light and dark colors, hard and soft surfaces, and smooth and rough textures.

In a study of seven breastfeeding support groups, the researchers were looking for reasons some support groups increased breastfeeding rates in attendees, while others didn't. Some reasons had to do with the environment: "Sensory aspects of the environment (appearance, light, comfort, smell, refreshments, temperature, and noise) were important..." "Place could negatively influence provider behavior...cold uncomfortable environments which were de-motivating to all" (Hoddinott, Britten, & Pill, 2010).

Notice the details of your workspace. Does the flicker of the overhead lighting give you a headache, or does that initial purple glow shock you when the switch is turned on? What is in your office that gives a lift to your spirit, makes you smile, or is a nice place to take a nap?

Wise mentors and experienced clinical supervisors have taught me to mother the mother, so she will mother her baby. A classic study in the doula literature speaks to this point: researchers in South Africa found that mothers who were talked to, smiled at, and stroked in labor were more likely to talk to, smile, and stroke their newborn babies (Sosa, Kennell, Klaus, Robertson, & Urrutia, 1980). Mothers receiving mothering in labor mothered their own babies better. Figure out a way to mother your client. Giving her something is one way. I have sometimes brought a head of green cabbage to a home visit with a new mother. It makes her laugh, and she can always eat it. A new mother's gut can always use the roughage!

If only a tissue or a carafe of spring water and a cup are available, give it to her to help her feel cared for and consequently more likely to engage in a therapeutic relationship. Meeting her physical needs is part of the therapeutic environment; water, a pretty glass, and a box of tissues are cheap to the pocket and nourishing to her spirit. When you remind her that healing takes time, you are helping her relax.

Where you sit in relation to the mother is part of the environment. There is a difference between standing over a person who is lying down in bed and sitting in a chair next to her bed. Sitting next to her communicates equality and a willingness to engage. A busy staff person can relax while sitting, and that relaxation communicates to the client. On rare occasions, intuition has led me to sit on the floor at a mother's feet and look up to her, as a way to help her feel valued and important.

Some women are too shy to experiment with new techniques in front of a stranger, even a gentle and loving one such as yourself. A new mother like this may enjoy a breastfeeding video or DVD to watch in the privacy of her own home. She can also benefit from watching streaming videos on the Web or www.youtube.com. Do a Google search of the topic yourself, so you know what she will find and what you will choose to recommend.

When your environment is comfortable and special in a way that speaks to you, it will nourish you and make you feel comfortable, so you can do your best work. When you take control over your internal environment, even if it is as small an action as taking three deep breaths between patient rooms, going to the toilet, or staring out the window for a minute, you will feel centered, calmer, and ready to meet the next patient. Pausing with your hand on a doorknob and taking a deep breath before opening the door gives you some control over the energy of the day. Those ten-second pauses are little refreshing breaks. They are something you can give to yourself. If you don't take care of yourself, who will?

Environment creates the space for healing work. It is particularly important in lactation therapy and in helping the wounded dyad recover breastfeeding.

Connecting the Dots between Birth and Breastfeeding

Breastfeeding difficulties can have their origin in labor, delivery, and birth.

Human Patterns of Birth Are Culturally Shaped

Birth and breastfeeding have evolved (or been created, depending on one's personal beliefs) as successful strategies for human propagation. An increase of four billion humans in 60 years—from 2.8 billion in 1950 to 6.8 billion in 2010—proves the success[16] of the human biologic template for reproduction.

There are a few universal truths for all things human. One is that humans gather in groups: families, clans, tribes, parishes, religious or ethnic groups, professional and work associations, and countries. My esteemed colleague, Chris Mulford, RN, BSN, and IBCLC, has said that culture is, "what we know and what we do that makes us part of a group." Every group has its own culture, its own customs and arts, social institutions and achievements, unique views and beliefs, and ways of living. While the physiologic elements of pregnancy, birth, and breastfeeding are similar for every woman, culture shapes the environment and conduct of childbearing.

What is the natural, undisturbed physiologic pattern, the biologic template of human childbearing? No one knows for certain, although many (psychologists, feminists, philosophers, physicians, anthropologists, and more) have offered scholarly opinions. Other mammal species, such as dogs, fruit bats, and marmosets, have similar courtships, pregnancies, labors, births, breastfeeding, and weaning, no matter where they live. Humans do not. Should women be left alone in labor, be in the company of trusted, knowledgeable female companions, or be drugged and confined to bed and monitored by machines and licensed strangers? When and for how long should the baby be breastfed? Practices are different, depending on where the mother and baby live.

16   http://www.census.gov/ipc/www/idb/worldpopgraph.php

Culture and Breastfeeding

Dr. Katherine Dettwyler has studied weaning patterns of other mammals, including primates, to use scientific reasoning to extrapolate the length of human breastfeeding. Culture has such an impact on infant feeding practices that global human weaning ages range from the day of birth to a rumored 13 years, although UNICEF does not go beyond 20 to 23 months in its recordkeeping, and the 13-year figure is an ephemeral image.[17] Dr. Barbara Rogoff (2003), after reading a paper written about 52 societies, suggested a range of six months to five and one-half years, with two and one-half years in the middle.

Dr. Dettwyler (Dettwyler & Stuart-Macadam, 1995) explored the correlation of weaning age with life history variables in primates, as reported by a number of researchers on the topic. Some of the life history variables associated with primate weaning are: the quadrupling of infant birthweight, eruption of first adult teeth, when the infant reaches one-third of the adult female weight, or six times the length of gestation. Based on those parameters, Dr. Dettwyler speculated that "most humans would be weaned somewhere between two and one-half and seven years of age" (Dettwyler & Stuart-Macadam, 1995, p. 66).

Contrast this two-and-one-half to seven-year range with the CDC's (2010a) latest figures of how many babies are exclusively breastfed for six months in the U.S. (about 13% in 2007), and how many babies are breastfeed for at least a year (18.5% in 2009; CDC, 2010b). Information about how many babies are breastfeeding for longer than one year of age is difficult to find. An informal poll run by the website, Parents Place, in 1998 revealed that 6% of babies nursed past the second year.[18] A formal survey of 179 mothers in La Leche League found that 66% were nursing at age two; the range of weaning in this sample was six months to seven years, with the average between two and one-half and three years (Sugarman & Kendall-Tackett, 1995). The sample surveyed was all La Leche League members, a group likely to breastfeed a long time.

The most recent CDC reports for 2007 show that while breastfeeding initiation is up, exclusivity and duration have declined since 2006. This is the wrong direction!

There are many reasons for the breastfeeding rates that are below the Healthy People 2020 goals for the U.S. One is the reliance on technology to manage birth. Another is that "birth facilities in most states are not

---

17   http://www.childinfo.org/breastfeeding_iycf.php
18   http://www.kellymom.com/writings/bf-numbers.html#various

providing maternity care that is fully supportive of breastfeeding" (CDC, 2010c). The mother and baby rarely get to meet in an environment that supports mutual exploration and falling in love. There are insufficient numbers of hospital staff. Not all staff understands, respects, and supports breastfeeding. The unrestrained presence in hospitals of the formula industry (with its sales force, free samples, and free supplies) is another significant barrier to breastfeeding.

When labor and birth are managed by technology, breastfeeding can suffer. The difficulty lies sometimes with the mother, sometimes with the baby, and other times with both. Occasionally, the difficulty lies in the breast or with the milk production. A dyad can face more than one challenge.

Pregnancy and Birth Today

Reliance on technology reflects a reductionist or mechanistic viewpoint. If a machine stops running, then each part is evaluated. When the parts are all working well, the machine functions efficiently. How machines *feel* about their work doesn't matter; whereas, how a mother feels about her labor, her breasts, and her baby matters very much. Common maternity care practices today rely on time limits, laboratory results, and machine readouts more than they do on the mother's feelings and inherent biological processes.

Routine standard obstetrical care requires each mother to be thoroughly scrutinized at each prenatal visit. She has her blood tested, her baby visualized with ultrasounds (as many as ten over the course of the pregnancy, depending on her insurance plan), she is monitored for a variety of diseases and conditions, and the condition of her cervix is checked with a pap smear. She also receives regular measurement of her weight, blood pressure, urine protein and sugar, uterine growth, and baby's activity. She is given warnings about food and drink, medications and drugs, vitamins, Vitamin D, cat litter boxes, environmental hazards, and infectious diseases. A pregnant mother may work full-time right up to labor, so as to have maximum maternity leave; she may start labor already tired. Living pregnant while undergoing constant surveillance "to be sure things are okay" does not build self-confidence.

Obstetrical providers, who used to rely on their eyes and ears and hands for assessment, now rely on tests and machines. Two examples illustrate how reliance on test results or machine readings conflict with direct experience. A mother pregnant with her third baby (after two full-term gestations and normal vaginal deliveries) told her obstetrician that her baby had dropped (engaged in her pelvis) at the 36-week prenatal visit. Instead of believing the voice of experience, or looking at the woman's belly to confirm the fetal position and altered abdominal profile, or palpating the fetal position, the obstetrician sent the mother for an ultrasound. It would have been much cheaper if the obstetrician had used hands and eyes instead of an expensive (and potentially risk-inducing) machine. A hands-on examination would have been convenient, and some discussion would have occurred during the examination–a splendid opportunity for teaching!

The second example is a cliché where the first-time laboring mother says, with great urgency, "the baby is coming now," and the maternity staff replies, "Oh no, you have a long way to go yet, dearie; it's only your first time." Then the baby slides out in the labor bed. This is a cliché because it is so common. Some experiences are undeniable, even when never before experienced, such as the baby coming out. Yet the mother is often the last person to be believed, despite the fact that she is the one actually having the experience.

Machines and medications play a major role in most hospital labors. As a labor and delivery nurse following physicians' orders on maternity units in the 1990s, I administered a certain number of drops per minute of IV fluid with ten units of Pitocin™ in it, and increased the number of drops per minute until the mother was having three contractions in ten minutes, each contraction lasting for one minute. Audiences of hospital staff attending my lectures have brought the phrase "pit to distress" to my attention. This means that the Pitocin™ infusion rate is increased until the baby's heart rate indicates the baby is getting distressed, whereby an emergency cesarean section can be justifiably performed. A Google search of the phrase in February 2011 yielded over one million hits.

I've witnessed hospital staff discount a woman's experience of her own labor, saying, "You aren't having strong contractions now, the monitor isn't showing anything." The fetal monitor is considered more reliable than the woman's perceptions. It is possible to do nearly all the physical assessment using probes, strain gauges, IV lines, and monitor leads. There is little need to touch the patient with bare hands. Newborns are touched with probes (scalp leads), silicon vacuum cups, steel forceps, and gloved hands, as per policy. Patients are bathed by nursing staff wearing gloves.

The evidence shows that women touched, smiled at, and talked to in labor are more likely to touch, smile at, and talk to their new babies than women receiving standard care (Sosa et al., 1980). Laboring women who are mothered, who are not talked to, smiled at, or touched will be less engaged with their babies. Hospital staff walking into the room where a woman is laboring go to the machines first to see what is happening; rarely do they engage with the mother first. This model of disengagement may be influencing how the woman will mother her new baby. How will a woman feel about breastfeeding if she is less engaged with her baby?

A mother's confidence is like a bud; hospital teachings and practices can blight that bud so it doesn't bloom. What happens to a new mother's confidence that she can keep her baby alive when she is given a crib card that it is a list of warnings about infant safety? Along with advice to put her baby on its back for sleep and to ask to see staff identification before letting the baby leave the mother's room, the card says, "Do not carry the baby in your arms in the hospital. Push the baby in the crib."

I feel strongly that some of the uncertainty and insecurity I see in my office comes from these hospital dicta, born of risk management and fear of liability in case of a fall. Mothers readily carry grocery bags, laundry, and pets; yet, they are unsure about carrying their own babies. How can a mother relax enough to let her milk flow when she has learned that carrying her baby is dangerous? How else could more than one new mother ask the question, with deepest sincerity, "How do I hold my baby?"

U.S. Birth Statistics

The CDC (2010c), in the Maternity Practices in Infant Nutrition and Care 2007 survey, discovered that "a substantial proportion of (maternity) facilities used maternity practices that are not evidence-based and are known to interfere with breastfeeding." Some of these practices are medical intervention and over-use of technology in labor, insufficient staff training, antiquated policies, and routine separation of mother and baby. Current statistics give a picture of the state of birth in the U.S.

How often is labor and birth technology used in the U.S.? In a representative sample of women who gave birth in 2006, 57% received synthetic oxytocin (Pitocin™) to speed or induce labor, 94% had continuous electronic fetal monitoring used throughout labor, 57% delivered lying on their backs, 83% received intravenous fluids, and 76% used epidural or spinal anesthesia (Sakala & Corry, 2008).

The U.S. rate of labor induction has more than doubled since 1990. According to ACOG, in 2006, more than one woman in five had her labor induced.[19] Different surveys will yield different results. With respect to inductions, all the numbers are too high.

When my first baby was born in 1975, the national cesarean section rate was 12%. In 2008, the national cesarean section rate was 32.3%, the 12th

19 www.choicesinchildbirth.org/resource/CIC_2011_Philadelphia_BirthGuide_WebMech_01_hires.pdf

year of a consecutive yearly increase (USDHHS, 2010). Regional rates vary, with some hospitals in my region (Philadelphia, PA, USA) having cesarean section rates over 40% in 2008 (USDHHS, 2009a).

The World Health Organization states that an acceptable cesarean section rate is ten to 15% (WHO, 1985). Some researchers believe that more harm than good occurs when the cesarean section rate rises over 15% (Althabe & Belizan, 2006). Health organizations around the world, where other countries, such as Brazil, have cesarean section rates over 50%, are vociferous in their concern over the increase in surgeries (Zhang et al., 2008).

Cesarean section has a negative impact on the hormones of lactation. Swedish researchers discovered that prolactin levels and oxytocin pulsatility were lower on day two postpartum after a cesarean section (Nissen et al., 1996). Breastfeeding and lactogenesis are affected when breastfeeding hormone activity is low; there is a delay in the onset of milk volume increase (Evans, Evans, Royal, Esterman, & James, 2003). Breastfeeding is more difficult because the baby may not get enough milk. Hospital staff then becomes concerned about the baby's weight loss, the mother catches their fear and her confidence in breastfeeding is undermined.

When a cesarean section is scheduled, the baby is removed without labor and has no warning or preparation for life outside the womb. Babies born by cesarean section without labor are at risk of respiratory distress (Sotiriadis, Makrydimas, Papatheodorou, & Ioannidis, 2009). Babies born with breathing difficulty will not breastfeed and are taken away from their mothers for specialized care. Separation is another barrier to the establishment of breastfeeding.

When breastfeeding is difficult, the mother worries. Worry interferes with milk-related hormone release, which makes breastfeeding more problematic, which increases the worry, and so on *ad infinitum*. Worry stimulates the release of adrenalin and stress hormones like cortisol. Stress hormones impede the milk-moving hormones, so her milk won't flow. The baby goes to breast and is frustrated. The mother's breasts harden and hurt, as they swell with milk that can't flow. The baby has more trouble attaching to a swollen breast, less milk is removed, the breast gets fuller, and a vicious cycle develops.

The use of machines and interventions is associated with a delay in the onset of Lactogenesis II, milk volume increase, referred to in the vernacular as the "milk coming-in" (Grajeda & Perez-Escamilla, 2002; Dewey, Nommsen-Rivers, Heinig, & Cohen, 2003; Nommsen-Rivers & Dewey, 2009). Delay in milk volume increase contributes to infant weight loss. Nommsen-Rivers and Dewey (2009) discovered that the infant cohort in two affluent cities in California had more infants lose excessive amounts of weight in the first week of life when compared with similar cohorts in Italy and Peru. The authors state, "Childbirth is a highly medicalized event in the United States, and this type of birth setting may contribute to additional challenges in successfully establishing lactation."

The consequences of the routine use of birth technology go beyond the immediate postpartum period. There is an impact on society, too: high rates of cesarean section (CDC, 2010d), high rates of prematurity (12-13%) compared with five to nine percent in other developed nations (Goldenberg, Culhane, Iams, & Romero, 2008), and PTSD and depression in mothers (Alcorn, O'Donovan, Patrick, Creedy, & Devilly, 2010; Simkin, 1991; Creedy, Shochet, & Horsfall, 2001; Rowe-Murray & Fisher, 2001). Routine birth technology increases healthcare expenditures and medical (hazardous) waste that is either burned or dumped, further stressing our precious and limited global environment.

Impact of Induction

The CDC reported in 2004 that one out of every eight infants was born preterm, and in 2010 that 42% of preterm singleton infants were born without spontaneous labor, either by induction or by cesarean section (MacDorman et al., 2010). These statistics are now being integrated into public health education campaigns—high rates of prematurity are a public health concern.

The way preterm babies are managed has changed over the course of my clinical career. As a nursing student in the early 1970s, I was taught that babies had to be feeding well, be at least 37 weeks gestational age, and weigh at least five pounds before they could be discharged from the hospital. Nowadays, babies weighing less than five pounds are sent home, some with gestational ages of 35 weeks! Early babies are so common that the Academy of Breastfeeding Medicine offers a protocol for Breastfeeding the Near-Term Infant, one that is 34 to 36-6/7 weeks gestational age.

Common does not mean normal. The induced newborn isn't ready to be out in the world. Breathing, dealing with gravity and changing temperature, and the abrupt halt of steady nourishment are challenging to a baby that needs a few more days or weeks inside to grow mature enough to be born. Near-term infants prefer sleeping to anything else, including breastfeeding.

Late pre-term births are becoming mainstream issues. A front-page article in *The Philadelphia Inquirer* on Monday, August 2, 2010, states "Near term' babies, not as sturdy as implied, have become a growing class of preemies," this article reflects growing public awareness of this problem.

The protocol for "Breastfeeding the Near-term Infant" recommends skin-to-skin care, unrestricted breastfeeding, and expression of newborn milk to be fed to the infant.[20] Dyads that meet after induction of labor require special care and intervention in this protocol to breastfeed with any success. Not every mother of a near-term infant is guaranteed this depth of care.

Long-Distance Relationships Are Difficult

In the U.S. in 2008, about one woman in three went home with a newborn and an abdominal incision. Most were separated from their babies during the hospital stay. Separation is more detrimental to breastfeeding than labor medication.

In the five counties surrounding Philadelphia, listed by the U.S. Census Bureau in 2009 as the sixth most populous city in the U.S., many hospitals routinely separate newborns from their mothers for up to four hours after delivery (Crivelli-Kovach & Chung, 2010). Hospital breastfeeding assistance is hit or miss. Hospitals lack enough staff proficient in basic breastfeeding management skills. Not all new mothers are given accurate guidance. If the lactation staff is unavailable, and the staff advice is inconsistent or inaccurate, the new mother doubts herself, her baby, and breastfeeding.

There is no evidence to support the practice of separating a healthy newborn from its mother at birth. No one has won the $1,000 I offer to any student in my classes who brings me a well-done study showing that it is beneficial to take healthy newborns away from their mothers. Lennart Righard and Margaret Alade (1990) discovered in 1990 that only seven babies out of 34 had correct suckling if they had been taken away from their mothers after birth for only 20 minutes. Twenty-four babies out of 38 had correct suckling if left on their mothers' torso, skin-to-skin until the first breastfeed.

Klaus and Kennell (1982) describe the impact of post-birth mother-infant separation on maternal behavior; Odent (1999) speaks to this point, also. All these researchers documented that what was true for antelopes, sheep, goats, rats, hamsters, and monkeys was also true for humans, that maternal-infant separation is detrimental (in some species, even fatal) to the newborn mammal. Klaus and colleagues (1995), in a later work, present both evidence and case histories showing that the earlier and more frequent the contact, the more likely the mother is to keep her baby with her. An

20   http://www.bfmed.org/Resources/Protocols.aspx

Australian study done in 2001 found an association between maternal depression at eight months postpartum and delayed contact with her baby at birth (Rowe-Murray & Fisher, 2001).

Kennell and Klaus (1998) have described the importance of the critical period after birth, saying, "Encouraging mother-infant contact from birth on and rooming-in could increase breastfeeding significantly and decrease the incidence of failure to thrive, abuse, neglect, and abandonment of infants." The research papers that support their observations would fill your car.

Anyone that has been in a long-distance romantic relationship knows that intimacy is difficult to maintain when the parties involved spend little or no time together. The breastfeeding relationship is no different. Achieving confidence and competence is difficult when mothers and babies start with a long distance relationship, far apart, with the baby in the nursery and the mother in her postpartum room. The American Academy of Pediatrics, in its breastfeeding policy statement, recommends keeping newborns in close physical proximity to promote breastfeeding. This should start in the hospital. Step 7 of the 10 Steps to Successful breastfeeding speaks directly to this point, advising all mothers to have 24-hour rooming-in.

The new mother has to assume all the properties of the placenta to ensure that her newborn will survive, including feeding and creating a safe environment. This is a scary, powerful, and necessary life passage. New mothers often worry that their baby may stop breathing, or get enough milk, or gain weight, or stay well (Stern, 1998). The new mother's openness to learning after delivery is a manifestation of this passage. As visual learning is the predominant mode for most humans, new mothers learn from what they see others doing (OSHA, 1996).

New mothers watch as hospital staff pushes wrapped babies around in wheeled carts. They never see a nurse carry a baby in arms. I've worked in hospitals where the policy was that infants could not be carried from one place to another; this is still true. Over the course of a clinical career, starting in 1971, I have noticed an increase in the numbers of mothers who do not carry their infants in arms, preferring instead to carry a large, awkward car seat in which the infant is strapped. I wonder if this is the result of early postpartum visual learning.

Weak Foundation, Weak House

The foundation for breastfeeding can be derailed in hospitals. One way is to give breastfed newborns formula. In 2008, 42% of breastfed babies received formula in hospital before two days of age (Grummer-Strawn, Scanlon, & Fein, 2008). Another study (Crivelli-Kovach & Chung, 2010) cites 80%. Both are beyond the 25% reported by the National Immunization Survey for 2007 births (CDC, 2010e).

Babies are supplemented with bottles of formula for a variety of reasons: because the mother lacks confidence, because staff doesn't believe that colostrum works or is sufficient, because the mother and baby are separated, because the staff member wants the baby to be quiet during the hearing or car seat test, because it has always been done that way, because the baby is in the nursery at night, because the grandmother wants to feed the baby, and because many (parents and staff alike) believe that "one bottle won't hurt." The evidence is overwhelming that all these practices interfere both with breastfeeding and with milk making. There seems to be an ongoing battle for who should feed the baby. Should it be the mother and her nurturing, species-specific milk? Or should it be everybody else (hospital staff, family) with human milk substitutes? Modern practice in hospitals too often favors the latter.

At a bare minimum, two practices need to be in place for breastfeeding to be successful. One is that mothers can breastfeed independently before they go home, and the other is that infants receive no formula (McCallister, Bradshaw, & Ross-Adjie, 2009). Breastfeeding independently means that mother can keep her baby close, notice early feeding cues, put her baby to breast, and let her baby feed and detach. Keep mother and baby together all the time in the hospital, so they learn what they need before they go home. Everything the newborn gets should be from mamma. This means heat, skin-to-skin contact, calming, love, and perfect nutrition.

Impediments to Breastfeeding

In many maternity units, there is a gap between historically driven clinical practice and current lactation knowledge. Fortunately, there is strong support from U.S. organizations (the CDC, DHHS, the Office of Women's Health, the Joint Commission, and the U.S. Breastfeeding Committee) that have launched campaigns, changed requirements, and funded public health surveys. This effort is spreading to the state and local levels, as precious grant monies are awarded for work in the breastfeeding field. Breastfeeding support is being integrated into more healthcare professional training programs. In January 2011, Surgeon General Regina Benjamin released a Call to Action to Support Breastfeeding, suggesting 20 actions to improve breastfeeding initiation, exclusivity, and duration. The momentum is building for the U.S. to be a nation where babies breastfeed wherever they are and no one notices, and where rates of pediatric diabetes and obesity are so low that everyone notices.

Much has happened to boost breastfeeding during my clinical career. In 1986, there were only two videos available for teaching, one from La Leche League and one from Kittie Frantz, RN, CPNP-PC. Now many new ones are released yearly. Breastfeeding articles used to be challenging to find; breastfeeding professionals traded copies with each other like baseball cards. Now there are at least four journals devoted to breastfeeding, in addition to articles published in every type of journal. It is so much fun to see the world open up to breastfeeding.

With all that momentum and zest, there are also dedicated and concerned healthcare practitioners who do not enjoy the information explosion about breastfeeding. Such people may not be so current, nor that respectful of breastfeeding, or they may have had a personal experience that was awful, and teach from their own history. They may believe that there isn't much to learn about breastfeeding since they received their fundamental education, and continue practices that are less than helpful.

Such an unfavorable practice is the guidance known as R.A.M., an acronym for Rapid Arm Movement. This technique that became popular in the 1990s when Chloe Fisher, the wonderful British midwife, was filmed telling a mother, "Wait for his mouth to open… wait… wait… NOW, whiz him on!" as she used the mother's arm to push the baby quickly towards the breast.

Ms. Fisher taught this technique in conferences, books, and videos. It spawned a variety of forced practices that staff, lacking any instruction in breastfeeding management, taught to each other and to mothers.

Clients have described to me how a hospital staff member took their breast in one hand and the baby in the other, and shoved them together, part A (nipple) into part B (infant mouth). I've heard peers brag that they could get any baby to latch on, no matter what the circumstance. Another forced technique is described as "screw in the light bulb," where the back of the baby's head is pushed forward, pushing the baby's face (with a hopefully opened mouth) onto the nipple. Sometimes a staff person will take the mother's nipple and massage the baby's lips with it, hoping to elicit rooting. Some mothers work so hard to make the baby grasp the breast that once the baby has latched on, they freeze in position, fearing the baby will let go. Others hold the baby's head so tightly at the breast that the baby fusses and squirms in protest. Mothers can interpret this fussing as the baby rejecting their breast or not liking breastfeeding. Sometimes babies fight the breast when the forced technique is used, then the mother increases her force to make the baby breastfeed; the end result is a battle.

Once home, a baby that has had its head rammed onto the breast often enough may either refuse to breastfeed or breastfeed in a way that hurts or injures the mother. Diane Wiessinger, MS, IBCLC, commented at a health provider conference that lactation consultants are teaching mothers to "dominate and control their babies' (breast) feeding" (Wiessinger, 2009). She postulates that the rise of formal breastfeeding management has further removed breastfeeding from its physiologic template. R.A.M. is an example of such domination.

I am amazed whenever I hear someone today, either client or healthcare professional, describe using R.A.M. As a routine practice, it is obsolete. It would be better to think of it as a tool in the breastfeeding helper's toolbox, used only in the most rare and specific circumstances. Chloe Fisher herself has said that the breastfeeding helper should only assist with breastfeeding by handling the breast when all else has failed. Forced techniques ignore infant readiness, signaled by feeding cues and primitive neonatal reflexes. The baby must grasp the breast with its mouth and hands; the nipple *cannot* be stuffed into the baby's mouth as the baby will move its tongue to block the invasion.

The reliance on the clock to regulate breastfeeding is another impediment. Hospital staff may advise mothers that the baby MUST feed every two or three hours. This dictum is fueled by healthcare professionals fearing they will be held liable should the baby be readmitted for dehydration or jaundice, from lack of knowledge about infant abilities, from a fundamental mistrust of early breastfeeding, and by long tradition of feeding babies by the clock. Hospital staff will tell mothers to "breastfeed on cue, every two to three hours." In other words, feeding a baby on cue is fine, as long as the baby cues within the recommended interval. What do new mothers do with this confusing advice? How can they reconcile what they are told with what their babies do?

If her baby doesn't wake to feed at the prescribed interval or wants to feed several times in a short interval, mothers can doubt their milk supply or their baby. Why should a baby that has been feeding continually while inside the womb be expected to feed at precise, fixed intervals? Why is a healthy baby assumed to lack the wherewithal to ask to eat? Healthy babies can be trusted. Keep mother and baby together, so they can communicate with each other and build their own unique relationship.

A mother who demands a feeding schedule or who becomes anxious and upset when the baby goes off schedule may be saying she is insecure or needs more information about newborn language and behaviors. Some mothers decide to set their alarm clocks to ring every two or three hours during the night, so they can wake up and, in turn, wake their sleeping newborns, and make them breastfeed RIGHT NOW. A baby wakened thus from deep sleep has no desire to eat. The baby will refuse to breastfeed, will grasp the breast in a way that hurts or injures the mother, or will breastfeed poorly. The dyad may fight with each other at every feed, a battle at the breast that the baby always wins. The mother exhausts herself with the frequent night waking and is out of synchrony with her own and her baby's natural rhythms. The baby is equally miserable. The saddest result is premature weaning and a mother who discourages her friends from breastfeeding because her own experience was so awful.

When they sleep together, it makes life easy. The mother doesn't have to be awake for the baby to find the breast. The baby doesn't have to be awake to feed. Mothers that are exclusively breastfeeding can be encouraged to explore safe bed-sharing options. At the very least, the baby should be in the bedroom. Mothers could also consider a side-car sleeping arrangement—a separate surface attached to her bed.

Many women are isolated and exhausted trying to keep to a pre-determined schedule, worried their baby will starve to death if they don't. Some wean or start pumping and bottle-feeding saying, "I'm going back to work in a few months, so I might as well get used to pumping now." Infant feeding becomes a dreaded chore instead of being integrated into life and becoming a sweet relationship. Integration of breastfeeding into her life is important because mothers have to be able to breastfeed while doing other things for breastfeeding to last for a long time. This is a reason I teach mothers to stand while breastfeeding.

Hospital staff sometimes complains that mothers from other cultures will not breastfeed in the first few days, citing "no milk." Yet, when a baby is jaundiced or hypoglycemic, the first response from staff in many facilities is to give the baby formula. Hospital staff don't believe in newborn milk (aka colostrum) either! Does a new mother believe what she is told (breastfeed), or what she sees the experts doing (giving her baby a bottle of formula)? How many of us remember being told as children, "Do what I say, not what I do?" Did it make any sense?

A mother from Zanzibar, a country where breastfeeding is routine, described her hospital experience, "My baby was given formula in the nursery against my wishes. It made my baby so sick that she had to go to the Intensive Care Nursery. The doctor tested *my* milk to see if it was making my baby sick." The safety of the formula was never questioned; the possibility that the formula was making the baby sick was never considered.

Formula supplementation in the postpartum unit undermines the mother's commitment to breastfeeding; why should she breastfeed if the healthcare worker, the one with the white coat and the authority, the expert, is giving formula to her baby? If the health worker is giving her an industry-branded diaper bag containing coupons and free samples of formula as she is going home, again, why should she breastfeed? The gift bag tells the family, as well as the mother, that infant formula is okay. Telling the new mother that the formula sample is there "just in case" undermines confidence in breastfeeding by introducing doubt. Worry makes breastfeeding more difficult.

The presence of formula sales representatives on maternity units contributes to a flat-line in U.S. exclusive breastfeeding rates. One of the Healthy People 2020 goals is that 44.3% of newborns be exclusively breastfed for the first three months of life; few states reached this objective in 2007, with the U.S. national average being about 33% (CDC, 2010e).

The Birthing Environment, Energy, and Emotion

Labor, delivery, and postpartum in U.S. hospitals is rarely undisturbed. Hospitals in the Philadelphia region have adopted a policy where a nurse must look in on each mother once an hour, day and night. Both mothers and nurses tell me they hate this; mothers, in particular, complain about being awakened at night, yet the practice continues.

One being watched perceives the watching. The reader has surely felt the sensation of being watched, perhaps as a student or as a child. A clever study measured skin conductance level (SCL) of subjects who were unaware of being observed. One subject stared at a live image of another subject on a video monitor, and the monitor was shut off at random intervals. Reliable changes in SCL, reflecting the monitor's on/off status, were noted in 66% of the subjects (Schlitz & LaBerge, 1997).

Privacy is essential for the oxytocin-releasing activities that revolve around reproduction: coition, gestation, and lactation. Internationally renowned Dr. Michel Odent speaks and writes about the mother's need for privacy during labor and birth. Humans usually seek privacy for intimate activities. Women need privacy and freedom from distractions to focus on what they need to do in labor and to initiate breastfeeding. Privacy is rare in most hospitals. Mothers are interrupted an average of 54 times in 12 hours on the first postpartum day by hospital staff and visitors (Morrison et al., 2006). How can a woman feel safe to bare her chest in such an environment?

The ease and quality of the breastfeeding relationship are an outcome of the ease of birth. The fabulous book, *The Impact of Birthing Practices on Breastfeeding*, compiles recent research connecting birth practices with breastfeeding and goes into far more detail than I can here (Smith, 2010). In over 35 years of my practice, there have been less than ten cases of lactation difficulty requiring a consultation when the birth was planned for and did occur at home. The greatest numbers of my clients have had hospital births, with Pitocin™ used in labor, along with an epidural. Many have endured induced labors and operative deliveries.

Mothers and babies both have unique sets of skills and reflexes to facilitate birth. Babies use the stepping reflex inside the uterus to propel themselves forward; the uterus has a pushing reflex, also called the fetal ejection reflex. The stepping reflex helps babies move themselves out of the womb. In most hospital births, babies rarely emerge from the womb in the physiologic way. Most commonly, babies are pulled out by their heads, or sucked out by a provider wielding steel instruments, a suction cup, or hands. This technology overrides the mother and baby's skills and reflexes. The only times I have ever seen a baby be pushed out naturally have been where the mother delivers before she gets to the hospital or at home births.

As the anatomy of the infant skull and the neck are designed to withstand being be pushed out, the external and unnatural force of pulling exerts more force on infant delicate structures, changing their dynamic relationship with each other. A baby can be injured when the pulling forces are exaggerated, as with a vacuum extractor or with forceps; bruising is obvious. Mothers have described their baby pulled so hard that they themselves slid down the table towards the physician. This frightens them because they imagine their baby being harmed. I have witnessed and heard tales of providers bracing their feet on the table to gain more pulling strength. The medical training video for the MightyVac™ vacuum extractor describes a built-in pop-off feature, where the vacuum will come off if the pressure goes too high. At the end of the film, there is a demonstration of how to over-ride the pop-off protective mechanism.

Using a vacuum extractor, or ventouse, carries risk to the infant's brain and spinal cord. The FDA issued an Advisory Warning about this device in 1998 (FDA, 1998). The vacuum was listed as a contributing cause of death to 12 infants and a cause of injury to nine, and concern was expressed for the level of technique currently in practice. Improper use of the vacuum led to brain bleeding. Dr. John Upledger, in his DVD, *Pediatrics: Treating Newborn Infants and Pregnant Mothers with CranioSacral Therapy,* likens the brain injury to a hickey, describing how the avulsed area becomes fibrotic.

Labor and delivery staff often asks a newly delivered woman if she wants her baby. This implies choice. The mother can either accept or refuse to see or hold her new baby. Could it be that staff asking if the mother wants her baby sends a message that time with a baby is optional and that it is all right to refuse, with the implication that mothering is a chore that can be delegated?

When biology suggests and evidence indicates that the best thing for the dyad to do after birth is to embrace each other and to breastfeed, presenting the meeting as an option, something that can be postponed, is not helpful. Sometimes hospital staff is overworked, as when there are cesarean sections back to back in the same operating room. When situations like this occur, there isn't always time for a lengthy first meeting, and the baby is with the mother only briefly before being taken away, thus shortening that precious first meeting. If the evidence were taken seriously, every new baby would be put on its mother's bared chest. She would be told, "Your baby has to be near your heart to recover from birth."

A breastfeeding relationship can start accidentally when the baby put skin-to-skin crawls to breast and starts feeding. Some mothers then change their feeding plans, saying, "Well, if breastfeeding is that easy, I think I'll do it." or "Wow, if she wants it that much, I guess I will do it." This is due in part to the inherent abilities and innate appeal of the newborn, and in part to maternal hormones, particularly prolactin and oxytocin. Widstrom and colleagues (1990) documented that mothers whose babies' mouths had touched the bare nipple or areola after birth, kept their babies with them longer.

New mothers sometimes say, "Take it away" or "eeuw" at the first sight of their new baby. I will always remember the wife of an obstetrical attending physician who told the nursing staff after a scheduled cesarean section that she didn't want to see her baby for at least 24 hours. Imagine a bride and groom, unwilling to see each other alone for 24 hours after the ceremony! When a mother is encouraged to leave her new baby to the care of strangers, falling in love and creating a bond becomes more difficult.

A new mammal mother is naturally curious about, interested in, and protective of her newborn. Could it be that a mother rejecting her newborn at birth signifies a serious disruption in the relationship and a disturbance with the emotional and energetic milieu necessary for breastfeeding? Could this disruption be considered a side effect of technologically driven birth?

After a baby is born, the practitioner goes on to the next case; the family goes home to pick up the pieces. Here is a client's birth story told to lactation consultant Jeanne Rago, BA, IBCLC, FILCA; details have been changed to protect privacy.

"A healthy primipara at 41 weeks gestation was told at a prenatal visit to go straight to the hospital for induction. The baby was fine, with a reactive heart rate, as measured during a non-stress test. The only reason for the obstetrician's alarm was that the pregnancy had gone one week past the estimated date of confinement. After 22 hours in bed with electronic fetal monitoring belts in place, without food, and given only ice chips for thirst, labor had not started, despite the use of Cervidil™ and hours of intravenous synthetic oxytocin, Pitocin™. The mother was given a 12-hour break to eat, sleep, and shower, and the induction resumed the next morning.

The second round of induction did not stimulate labor after six hours. The obstetrician then put a finger through the mother's cervix to separate the bag of waters from the interior wall of the uterus. When this didn't start labor after four hours, the bag of waters was broken. Regular contractions followed with subsequent cervical effacement and dilatation to one centimeter. After more hours of intravenous Pitocin,™ the mother was given an epidural. By the 70th hour of induction, her cervix was dilated to 10 centimeters, but her baby was not yet descended. The mother then pushed for three hours. The baby never descended. The obstetrician said that it was time for a cesarean section.

The baby was born healthy; the father went with the baby to the nursery to watch the routine infant admission procedure. When he returned to the recovery room, he found his wife writhing in pain with a "mob of hospital staff" surrounding her, one "jumping" on the top of her uterus, which was full of clots formed from the extended high doses of Pitocin™. No amount of morphine relieved her pain. The clots were removed and she was given medicine to control the bleeding. She was discharged home with hemoglobin of seven grams, but had not received a transfusion because the doctor felt that she looked "okay."

On postpartum day six, the parents brought the baby for breastfeeding help. They took turns narrating their story and weeping. They were stunned at the loss of all their dreams of a natural and spontaneous birth and easy breastfeeding. The mother had no confidence in her mothering, in her milk-making ability, nor her breastfeeding capacity. The father was overwhelmed by his helplessness. The baby had been fed bottles of formula in the hospital, another blow for this family."

When a family who is hurt and injured, in shock, with a baby that will not or cannot suckle effectively, come for breastfeeding help, there is a lot to heal, both for the caring practitioner who must deal with personal reactions to such stories, and for the family. Complementary and alternative therapies and soft technique provide a gentle, non-invasive approach that is well received.

When the fundamental connection between mother and baby is disturbed or disrupted in the hospital, outcomes vary. An article about 52 mothers who had planned to breastfeed describes two different paths that the mothers followed. This phenomenological study from New Zealand, where 34% of new mothers sampled reported going through a traumatic birth, identified these two paths as either struggling to sustain breastfeeding or giving up after too many barriers were encountered. Themes leading to sustained breastfeeding were: "proving oneself as a mother, sheer determination to succeed, making up for an awful arrival and atonement to the baby, and helping to heal mentally…" Themes leading to the abandonment of breastfeeding were: "just one more thing (the mother's breasts) to be violated, enduring the physical pain and seeming at times an insurmountable ordeal, the dangerous mix of birth trauma and low milk supply, intruding flashbacks and stealing anticipated joy, and disturbing detachment" (Beck & Watson, 2008).

The consequences of routine technology can be disastrous for breastfeeding, proving as challenging for the practitioner as for the dyad. This justifies using every bit of wisdom from every discipline available, so the mother-infant relationship and breastfeeding flourish. Complementary and alternative therapies, skin-to-skin care, remedial co-bathing, acupuncture, homeopathy and craniosacral therapy all have a role to play in breastfeeding, as will be presented in following chapters.

Mother-Friendly Childbirth and Baby Friendly Hospital Initiatives: Hope for the Future

Hospitals should and can be places where mothers are supported to labor free of unnecessary intervention, where breastfeeding is the norm, where mothers and babies are kept together, and where industry has no part in practice.

The Coalition to Improve Maternity Services developed the Mother-Friendly Childbirth Initiative in the 1990s as a designation for birthing facilities. The 10 Steps of the Mother-Friendly Childbirth Initiative means that a Mother-Friendly birth facility gives laboring mothers freedom to eat, move about, and have emotional and physical support from companions of their choice; to have sensitive and culturally appropriate care; to have the information necessary to make an informed choice about labor management; to be free from practices and procedures that are unsupported by scientific evidence; and to have breastfeeding promoted and supported by the WHO-UNICEF 10 Steps to Successful Breastfeeding.[21]

The World Health Organization and UNICEF developed the Baby-Friendly Hospital Initiative (BFHI) in 1991. Birth centers and hospitals that earn the Baby-Friendly designation are places where breastfeeding is helped and encouraged. There are about 20,000 hospitals with this designation in the entire world. Only 105 of them are in the U.S.[22]

The Baby Friendly Hospital Initiative incorporates maternal-infant contact as essential within its core, the 10 Steps to Successful Breastfeeding. Each step of the 10 Steps has a boatload of evidence supporting it.

Several of the steps are specific about early maternal-infant contact, skin-to-skin care, and keeping mothers and newborns together. Step 4 states, "Help all mothers to initiate breastfeeding within an hour of birth." Mothers are advised to hold their babies with skin contact, and to receive help from trained staff in order to initiate breastfeeding (WHO, 1998).

Step 7 says, "Practice rooming in–that is, allow mothers and babies to stay together–24 hours a day" (WHO, 1998, p. 62). To facilitate a strong mother-infant relationship, they have to be together as much as possible. For breastfeeding to become well established, they have to be in close contact as much as possible. There is no evidence to support routine nursery care, where newborns are away from their mothers. Studies going back to 1951 identify a strong association between rooming-in and improved breastfeeding outcomes (WHO, 1998, p. 62).

One study where the rates of infant abandonment were greatly diminished by the 10 Steps to Successful Breastfeeding was done in Russia. Rates of infant abandonment were cut nearly in half in the six years after Baby-Friendly practices were implemented (Lvoff, Lvoff, & Klaus, 2000). Contact promotes relationship; when relationship is established, love and attachment flourish, and the mother takes the baby home.

Increased breastfeeding is an outcome for Baby-Friendly hospitals everywhere in the world. At Boston Medical Center, breastfeeding rates increased to 87% (from 58%) once the BFHI was implemented. In U.S.-born African American women, breastfeeding rates rose to 74% (from 34% prior to BFHI implementation; Philipp et al., 2001). Mothers who didn't room-in, who weren't helped to breastfeed or sustain lactation when

---

21   www.motherfriendly.org/index.php
22   www.babyfriendlyusa.org

separated from their infants, whose babies received bottles of formula and pacifiers, and who were cared for by untrained staff at a facility with no breastfeeding policy were almost eight times more likely to discontinue breastfeeding before their babies were six weeks old (DiGirolamo, Grummer-Strawn, & Fein, 2001).

The Baby Friendly Hospital Initiative is becoming more popular and is recommended in the Surgeon General's Call to Action. It is both encouraging and helpful to have a specific set of strategies that work. One day, breastfeeding will be unquestioned in all maternity and newborn care practices.

Skin-to-Skin, Touch, and Breastfeeding

The Value of Touch

"More than any other human need, perhaps even more than food and shelter… we human beings need to touch one another" (Kornfield & Feldman, 1996).

Touch is powerful and life-sustaining for humans. The special touch of skin-to-skin contact between mother and baby is intimate, relationship-building, and a useful strategy in breastfeeding therapy. As the brain receives information through the eyes and ears, it also receives information through the skin. The eyes and ears interpret messages carried by light and sound; the skin interprets messages carried by touch.

The number of touch-related metaphors in language reflects its importance. Idioms and advertising slogans speak to the universality of touch. "Reach out and touch someone" was an advertising slogan for a telephone company. "He rubs me the wrong way" means that he annoys us. When something irritates us, it "gets under our skin." Sensitive people are considered to have "thin skin," whereas the insensitive are described as "calloused" or "thick-skinned." If we have to handle someone with "kid-gloves," it means they are tender or easily annoyed. Someone with the "Midas touch" turns things into gold, at least metaphorically. As lactation therapists, we wish for the "magic touch," the ability to help every mother and baby quickly and easily, and we "keep in touch" with mothers through telephone and email after the consultation to see how they are doing. In Spanish and Portuguese, playing an instrument is synonymous with touching it; the verb 'tocar' comes from the Latin 'toccare,' meaning 'to touch.'[23]

Baby mammals will grow up wild, unless they are touched enough. Owners of puppies are advised that touching, cuddling, and hugging a dog is important for socializing a dog into the world of people (Dunbar, 2011). Human babies are no different than any other mammal; they need touch to be socialized and to thrive.

Untouched human babies do not develop well. Romanian orphans, crowded into orphanages and deprived of tender, loving care, including touch, did

23   http://spanish.about.com/od/usingparticularverbs/a/using_tocar.htm

not grow nor acquire social skills or the ability for attachment. They were so neglected and deprived of contact that they lacked any emotional response to people (California State University, 2011). A professional colleague, visiting a Romanian orphanage, saw an infant that appeared to be about seven months old. When inquiry was made, my colleague was shocked to learn the baby was three years old!

Conversely, four-month-old infants, touched and held, along with other stimulation, showed more vocalization and smiling, and less crying (Field, 2002).

History of Touch

Touch is fundamental to humanity. Human history reflects the primal importance of touch.

The laying on of hands, the first recorded therapeutic touch, has been a method of benediction, comfort, and healing for all of recorded history. In both the Old and the New Testaments, the laying on of hands has signified blessing or granting authority, as when Isaac blessed his son Jacob (Genesis 27), when Aaron and the High Priests transferred the sins of the children of Israel to a sacrificial goat (Leviticus 16:21), and when priests were ordained. In the New Testament, the laying on of hands was linked to receiving the Holy Spirit (Acts 8:14-19). The Apostles laid hands on believers (Acts 6:5), and a bishop, priest, or minister would lay hands on the ill and weak, and pray for them to receive the Holy Spirit and be healed.

In Catholicism, anointing of the sick is the second sacrament of healing. The priest touches the sick or dying person with blessed oil for the purpose of healing or in farewell, as one of the Last Rites.[24] Eastern Orthodox and Eastern Catholic churches use blessed oil when laying on hands or ordaining clergy. The Anglican Church and the Latter Day Saints include the laying-on of hands to heal the sick, ordain an official, or confirm a new member.[25]

Members of royalty in England and France were thought to have the ability to cure skin diseases by virtue of being royal and possessing the Divine Touch. Kings Robert II the Pious, Clovis (Merovingian founder of the Holy Roman Kingdom), and Edward the Confessor laid their hands on the sick and the poor for healing. Queen Anne, in the early 1700s, was the last British royal to believe she possessed this divine talent. The French

---

24   http://en.wikipedia.org/wiki/Sacraments_of_the_Catholic_Church
25   http://en.wikipedia.org/wiki/Laying_on_of_hands

monarchy continued to believe and lay on hands at public holidays up to the French Revolution in 1789.

Diana, Princess of Wales, was a global icon for her entire adult life, starting with her marriage to the Prince of Wales in 1981. In 1987, she removed her gloves and extended her bare hand to a person with AIDS. This event made headlines in *Life Magazine* as the "Handshake seen around the world." She became the first celebrity photographed deliberately touching someone with an HIV infection.[26] Later on in her life, her personal crusade to ban land mines led her to be photographed embracing limbless children; her touch brought the world's eye to important topics, reinforcing universal humanity; her actions spoke louder than words.

The Untouchables are the lowest caste in India, although the term has been officially banned by constitutional law since 1950, and they since call themselves the Dalit. The life work of this lowest caste is jobs no one else will do, cleaning toilets and handling garbage. They are considered polluted, can pollute by their touch, and thus must stay away from everyone. In Meeting for Worship of the Religious Society of Friends (Quakers), we are asked to "hold" someone in the Light if they need special attention or healing. These are but a few of the many aspects of touch that are part of our lives, our thoughts, and our language.

Origins and Importance of Touch

Who knows when the different types of touch were named, or when tools (such as acupuncture needles or special oils) were invented to extend and augment touch? When was the intention in touch formalized into art and science, tradition, and schools? Perhaps the therapeutic use of touch was an outgrowth of the caressing and stroking, hugging and holding, and soothing and calming shared by mothers and their babies, and by lovers with their mates. Perhaps our primal memories include the sensations from the constant laving of our being while in utero, where we are safe, rocked, and warm. While gestating, all of a baby's cells are bathed and caressed by warm, moving liquid and tissue. The sense of touch is the earliest to develop in fetal life (Montague, 1986). By the beginning of the second trimester, babies are sensitive to touch, and will move away from the examiner's palpation of the mother's abdomen (Verny & Kelly, 1982; Klaus & Klaus, 1985).

Contact between the hands of the healer and the body of the person seeking healing is a welcomed strategy. Human touch makes our lives kinder and gentler. How many times has the reader heard a stressed friend or coworker say, "I just need a hug"? Contact between the layperson and the celebrity, strangers to each other, is valued as well; people will wait for hours after public events to shake the celebrity's hand.

Babies and mothers respond well to the warmth of human touch that conveys caring and acceptance. When breastfeeding is not going well, the relationship has a better chance of recovery when mother and baby get in touch with each other on all levels–physical and energetic. Skin-to-skin contact is one strategy that makes it easy for the dyad to become fascinated by each other.

Rachel Naomi Remen, MD, co-founder of the Commonweal Cancer Help Program and a Clinical Professor at the University of California San Francisco School of Medicine, writes about touch: "Like people with cancer, the doctors (*author's note: participants in a healing program run by Dr. Remen*) comment on how unusual it is to be touched by someone who only wants your well-being… They often comment that it would take only a simple inner shift to touch someone with a healing intent in the very process of doing a physical exam" (Remen, 1996). All the different styles of touch, and of the laying on of hands presented in this book, have healing intention in common.

Many hands-on therapies use a particular style of touch as the healing technique. This book will address ones with which the author is most familiar: skin-to-skin care, remedial co-bathing, massage, acupuncture, chiropractic, osteopathy, and craniosacral therapy. Some of these therapies are considered to be Complementary and Alternative Medicine (CAM); some are part of practice in hospitals and private offices. They are all variations of touch, useful as tools towards the goal of easy and comfortable breastfeeding.

The Skin

The skin is our largest organ and can be viewed as an external nervous system (Montague, 1986). The skin develops, along with sensory organs, from the ectoderm, the outer layer of the embryo. Six weeks after conception, the embryo will respond to touch, even before its eyes and ears have formed (Montague, 1986, p. 4). "As the most ancient and largest sense organ of the body, the skin enables the organism to learn about its environment. It is the medium… by which the external world is perceived" (Montague, 1986, p. 5). When a newborn mammal is skin-to-skin with its mother's ventral torso, it is in the perfect environment to find the breast.

Skin-to-skin stimulates and facilitates an infant's basic survival mechanisms, whether the baby is human, feline, or ursine.

Research About Skin-to-Skin Care for Preterm Infants

The value of skin-to-skin care for preterm infants has been the subject of extensive research, beginning in 1978 in Bogota, Colombia, with the work of Dr. Edgar Rey Sanabria, Professor of Neonatology in the Department of Pediatrics at the National University of Colombia. Dr. Sanabria looked for a way to keep low-birthweight babies alive in an environment characterized by overcrowding and a lack of resources (Charpak et al., 2005). His exploration and observation led to the formal practice known as kangaroo care or kangaroo mother care.

Several different terms are used to describe types of skin-to-skin care (SSC) between a mother and her premature baby. Kangaroo care and kangaroo mother care (KMC) are sub-sets of skin-to-skin care. KMC is defined as continuous skin-to-skin care, in which the mother wears her baby in a longitudinal lie between her breasts. The baby is nestled into a physiologically stable environment, much like a baby kangaroo that spends months cached in its mother's pouch, attached to her teat. In 1996, delegates at an international conference in Trieste, Italy, selected the term 'Kangaroo Mother Care' out of 30 terms in use at the time; the phrase means a program of skin-to-skin contact, exclusive breastfeeding, and early discharge. The term 'kangaroo care' refers to hospital skin-to-skin contact only. Since that time, as more people have become familiar with the concepts through many research articles, the terms have sometimes become synonyms of each other (Bergman, 2011).

In Colombia, KMC consistently reduced stress for mother and baby, and enhanced their bonding and the infant's growth, health, and development. KMC was integrated easily into the family environment and promoted breastfeeding. In 1999, the Kangaroo Foundation in Colombia was visited by the first of many delegations from India. These delegations, mostly nurses and doctors, return to India and start similar programs in their own locales (Bergman, 2011).

Mothers who had early skin-to-skin contact with their premature infants showed differences in attachment behavior for up to two years after delivery when compared with mothers whose first contact with their infants was three weeks after delivery (Kennell, Trause, & Klaus, 1975). Klaus and Kennell said, "For each species there seems to be a specific length of separation that can be endured. If separation extends beyond this sensitive period, the effects on mothering behavior are often drastic and irreversible" (Madrid & Pennington, 2000).

KMC is universally successful in improving infant survival. Reports from Madagascar (Ruize-Pelaez, Charpak, & Cuervo, 2004), Malawi, Brazil, Portugal (de Araújo, Rios, dos Santos, & Goncalves, 2010), and South Africa tell of its life-saving properties (Pattinson, Bergh, Malan, & Prinsloo, 2006). There are few modern-day hospital interventions with such a spectacular track record.

The Cochrane Collaborative meta-analysis speaks to the value of KMC in saving the lives of premature infants. Their plain language summary says, "Compared with conventional care, KMC was found to reduce severe illness, infection, breastfeeding problems, and maternal dissatisfaction with method of care, and improve some outcomes of mother-baby bonding" (Conde-Agudelo & Belizán, 2003).

Skin-to-skin care has an additional benefit; mothers make more milk for their premature babies after doing skin-to-skin care (Hurst, Valentine, Renfro, Burns, & Ferlic, 1997).

Readers interested in garments that hold babies in kangaroo position can find them available for purchase (see www.kangaroomothercare.com and www.preciousimagecreations.com for a link to products). The author has no personal or financial connection to these sites.

Research About Skin-to-Skin Care for Term Infants

The World Health Organization and the Cochrane Collaborative have done extensive meta-analyses of research about all forms of skin-to-skin care for mature infants. The WHO says: "… skin-to-skin contact between the mother and her baby immediately after birth reduces crying, improves mother-infant interaction, keeps the baby warm, and helps the mother to breastfeed successfully. No important negative effects were identified" (Puig & Sguassero, 2007).

The Cochrane Collaboration, after evaluating 30 studies involving 1,925 mother-infant dyads, states, "The intervention may benefit breastfeeding outcomes, early mother-infant attachment, infant crying, and cardio-respiratory stability, and has no apparent short or long-term negative effects" (Moore, Anderson, & Bergman, 2007). In 2009, the World Health

Organization and UNICEF issued a joint statement that identified skin-to-skin care as a way to keep the newborn warm (WHO & UNICEF, 2009).

Research validates the value of skin-to-skin as a life-saving strategy (Conde-Agudelo & Belizán, 2003), as a pain-relieving strategy, and as a way to promote maternal attachment (Evidence to Support the 10 Steps) and breastfeeding initiation and duration (Moore et al., 2007; Sinusas & Gagliardi, 2001; Moore & Anderson, 2007). Legendary researchers (including Ludington-Hoe, Cranston Anderson, Widstrom, Mattheissen, Christianssen, Klaus, Righard, and Alade to name but a few) have documented the ability of babies placed skin-to-skin with their mothers after birth to crawl to the breast and self-attach, just like any newborn kitten or pup.

What more needs to be said to convince anyone of the value of skin-to-skin care when the world's leading public health organization, the world's premier research collaboration, and an international body of physicians unanimously endorse it?

Impact of Touch on Human Development

Questions about the essential nature of humans have been recorded since the 5th century BCE in Egypt. The historian Herodotus tells the story of Pharaoh Psmatik I taking two newborns away from their families and giving them to a shepherd to be raised in isolation and silence. The impact of this upbringing on their personalities and social abilities was not recorded, although the children were said to have spoken an ancient tongue, older than that of the Egyptians. (The shepherd must have been unable to keep quiet.) Another experiment about nurturing contact in humans was documented by the historian Salimbene di Adam in his writings about King Frederick the Great in the 13th century. King Frederick was curious about language and wanted to know what language children would speak if they were not influenced by anyone speaking to them. Would the language of Adam and Eve be Latin or Greek or Aramaic, or would it be the language of the children's parents? Foster mothers and nurses that cared for the babies were forbidden to speak and to play with them. The experiment ended tragically; all the children died (Coulton, 1906).

In the 1500s, Mogul emperor Akbar the Great took babies from their parents before they could talk, and raised them for 12 years in an isolated castle, cared for by people who were deaf and mute. When these children were brought to the emperor, they could not speak. Again, history is silent about the adult lives of these children (Thomason, 2003). James IV of Scotland is said to have tried a similar experiment, with similar results.

In the beginning of the 1900s, German physician Martin Cooney used the newly invented incubator to keep premature infants alive. This was the first time in human history that a baby born too soon had a chance of survival. Dr. Cooney toured the world with the babies in their isolettes. At the 1932 World's Fair, the exhibition of his babies sold more tickets than any other except that of fan dancer Sally Rand. While premature infant survival rates were high, Dr. Cooney discovered that it was difficult for him to give the babies back to their mothers. The mothers were disconnected from the babies and not interested in having them back (Blum, 2002).

Skin-to-Skin Care at Birth Supports Breastfeeding

Nursing the newborn baby (or babies) after they are born is a universal characteristic of non-human mammals. The newly delivered mother positions herself to permit access to her teats; the newborns then wiggle, crawl, walk, or swim to the teat and suckle. Only in humans do cultural norms, values, and practices disrupt this basic mammalian template.

The neurochemical changes, the shifts and surges in essential hormones that occur in mothers and babies at birth are designed to ensure survival of the young through maternal giving of milk and love. Mothers and babies are primed to fall in love at birth because of the particular hormones that are released in labor and delivery. These hormones are essential at birth, both for the mother's recovery from the delivery process, for the initiation of breastfeeding, and for the mother and baby to become attached to each other and fall in love; a mother who loves her baby will take the best care of it.

The culturally recognized power of love and attachment hormones leads parents to keep adolescent girls away from adolescent boys because parents, knowing that adolescents are full of reproductive hormones, don't want particular behaviors to be acted out! Things are backwards here in the U.S.–we don't want our teens getting pregnant, and we want our babies to be breastfed. Yet our teens get together too often, and babies are routinely separated from their mothers after birth.

The evidence that supports the value of skin-to-skin care would float a boat to heaven. It is good for babies, premature or term. More babies go home with their mothers when there is immediate skin-to-skin care after birth (Step 4 of the BFHI) in Russia (Lvoff et al., 2000). It is good for mothers, as the skin-to-skin contact will make her shift into parasympathetic mode, with resultant increases in the mothering and milk-making hormones, oxytocin and prolactin, along with relaxation.

Dr. Nils Bergman, the South African neonatologist, speaks about "habitat-niche," pointing out that, depending on their environment, babies are in one of two modes: fight, flight, or freeze or grow and feed, depending on which part of their involuntary nervous system is activated–sympathetic or parasympathetic. Karl states that newborns rely on their caregivers to assist in regulating state and identifies babies who appear to be sleeping in the nursery as actually being in a state of "close down" or over-aroused; she suggests using skin-to-skin contact as a way to calm the over-aroused baby (Karl, 2004).

Our environment tells us how to behave and we respond to our perception of our environment. We learn about our environment through our senses. A newborn baby has highly developed tactile and olfactory senses. As breastfeeding is a blend of reflex behaviors (Colson, Meek, & Hawdon, 2008), the practitioner needs to create the environment that will elicit reflexes that will help the infant attach to the breast. We can't talk to babies and tell them to breastfeed. A baby can't function in a long-distance relationship. Being apart from the mother's body is long-distance to a newborn. Skin contact with their mothers is the ideal environment for the newborn.

In 2010, a prospective cohort study of 21,842 dyads born at 18 hospitals showed a dose-response relationship between skin-to-skin care after birth and breastfeeding exclusivity. This study (Bramson et al., 2010) replicates earlier work done in Guatemala (Klaus, Trause, & Kennell, 1975), Sweden (Widstrom et al., 1990), and Poland (Mikiel-Kostyra, Mazur, & Boltruszku, 2002). Both the Polish and California research is quantitative; the longer the baby spends skin-to-skin after birth, the more likely the mother is to breastfeed exclusively, and the longer she breastfeeds exclusively, the longer her breastfeeding duration.

Skin-to-skin care is recommended by the Academy of Breastfeeding Medicine in six of its 22 protocols: Hypoglycemia, Peripartum Management of the Term Infant, Model Hospital Policy, Breastfeeding the Near-Term Infant, NICU Graduate Going Home, and Breastfeeding the Hypotonic Infant (Academy of Breastfeeding Medicine, 2011) for thermoregulation of the infant and as a way to promote breastfeeding.

Babies, like all newborn mammals, can feed themselves from birth when put in the right environment, namely skin-to-skin on their mother's chest. Many women don't know this is possible, believing instead that they are 100% responsible for all of breastfeeding. This is a fallacy. The mother and the baby both have specific roles to play in the breastfeeding relationship. The mother has to provide the breasts and the milk, and keep the baby close to her heart. The baby has to latch on. Metaphorically speaking, the mother sets the table; the baby picks up the fork!

Skin-to-Skin Care in Breastfeeding Therapy

While skin-to-skin care at birth lays the foundation for breastfeeding, other research illuminates the value of skin-to-skin when breastfeeding has not been well established.

Skin-to-skin care puts the baby in the environment that is conducive to reflex self-attachment behaviors, provides a feeling of safety, and promotes physiologic stability and comfort. For the mother, skin-to-skin care can induce a hormonal shift favoring release of oxytocin, with the resultant improved connection between mother and baby. Harry Harlow said, "We believe that contact comfort has long served the animal kingdom as a motivating agent for affectional responses" (Harlow, 1958). Contact comfort restores the connection between mother and baby that may have never been well-established in the first few days postpartum, and one that may have been ignored in the subsequent days of recovery from birth injury and the work to establish a full milk supply.

Some mothers in my clinical practice have made comments at first visits such as, "He doesn't feel like my baby" or "I know she's mine, but I don't quite believe it" after labors and births that kept mother and baby separated after delivery, and when breastfeeding initiation has been delayed. These feelings are associated with breastfeeding difficulties. In such cases, skin-to-skin contact has opened the door to a positive change in maternal-infant connection and to breastfeeding. Putting the dyad literally in touch with each other is a useful strategy to strengthen or to restore their connection.

Using skin-to-skin care enabled mothers with breastfeeding difficulties to improve their breastfeeding (Chiu, Anderson, & Burkhammer, 2008). Skin-to-skin care facilitated breastfeeding for dyads having difficulties after birth; not only was breastfeeding made easier, but over half the dyads were exclusively breastfeeding at the one-month follow-up (Field, 2004).

Three case studies where skin-to-skin care was used for an hour before breastfeeding validate yet again the value of skin-to-skin care (Meyer & Anderson, 1999). Swedish midwife Kristin Svensson proclaims the value of putting a baby skin-to-skin and listening to the mother tell her story as a way to resolve breastfeeding difficulties. Her paper on this is awaiting publication (K. Svensson, personal communication, 2010).

Human mothers have the capacity to make an intellectual or moral commitment to a baby despite postnatal separation or traumatic birth. A mother will perform all the mothering tasks necessary to keep her baby alive and well tended out of intellect, will, societal expectation, and family support. For example, in the first few weeks after a cesarean section, Susan took her newborn to frequent specialist appointments (because of his multiple congenital anomalies), pumped both breasts eight times (for 15 minutes per session) in 24 hours, and attempted to breastfeed and bottle-fed her baby the collected milk. She also maintained the house, in addition to recovering from a cesarean section. Yet she never felt that Richard was "hers" until nearly four months postpartum after craniosacral therapy. (Susan and Richard will be discussed in more detail in the craniosacral therapy chapter.)

When mothers come for breastfeeding therapy, their history most frequently includes traumatic birth and separation. Mothers have told me of having their nursing baby removed from their breast because it was time to move from the delivery room to the postpartum ward, or of going for hours without seeing their new babies. In my region of the U.S., 56% of maternity hospitals separate newborns from their mothers for more than two hours, and 39% keep them apart for up to four hours (Crivelli-Kovach & Chung, 2010).

How to Integrate Skin-to-Skin Care into Clinical Practice

In the hospital or the private office, an ideal place to evaluate the breastfeeding relationship is with the mother and baby skin-to-skin. In the hospital, skin-to-skin assists the mother and baby to find each other for breastfeeding. In private practice, when things aren't going well, starting with skin-to-skin is helpful to see what the baby does and how the mother responds.

Once the baby is tucked in warmly on its mother's chest, then the practitioner and the mother can converse about the birth, about what has been going on, and about future plans, hopes, and dreams. On the postpartum ward, many times babies will crawl to the breast and self-attach while the mother is talking. The surprise on the mother's face when this happens is delightful. If, after being placed skin-to-skin, the baby goes into a deep sleep, then the mother can be taught how to hand express while the practitioner collects her milk in a spoon (there is always one on the food tray). Waiting for the mother to sigh or yawn, indicating a shift into parasympathetic mode, precedes easy milk flow.

Mothers sometimes feel completely responsible for the whole breastfeeding relationship. They are given instruction and handouts detailing the time intervals to feed, how to modify their environment, how to hold their breast and their baby, and how to latch their baby to the breast. All the instruction denies them any chance to explore and use their own instincts. In addition, they are too often in the presence of strangers and can feel awkward or shy about breastfeeding. In the hospital, some of my patients have said, "I'll feed my baby later, when the visitors have gone."

In such cases, giving the baby a chance to self-attach while in skin-to-skin contact shows the mother that her baby has the ability to feed. This gives the new mother tremendous relief and reinforces that breastfeeding is something that she and her baby do together.

Skin-to-skin care gives the mother a chance to experience her baby's ability to breastfeed, and gives the baby a chance to initiate interaction. When the baby does self-attach, a mother may feel a range of emotions. She can be amazed at her baby's ability. She can feel relief because the baby often latches on more comfortably and easier than when she was controlling everything. She can see that her baby wants her and wants to breastfeed. This is a healing experience; some mothers weep with surprise, joy, and pride.

How to Facilitate Breastfeeding in the Postpartum Ward

Knock on the door of the mother's room, introduce yourself, and request permission to enter. Suggest to the mother that the baby be brought into the conversation about breastfeeding. Tell her that putting the baby skin-to-skin, near the heart that it knows best, is bringing the baby into the conversation by giving the baby a chance to interact.

Close the door of the room AND pull the curtain around her bed. A closed door in a hospital is rarely taken seriously, and, often, staff comes barging in with no warning. A new mother may be reluctant to bare her breasts if she fears being interrupted. Pulling the curtain around her bed gives her a few seconds to cover herself should anyone suddenly enter the room.

Respect her new role as mother; she determines what will be done with or to her baby. Ask permission to touch or undress her baby. Offer her the option of undressing the baby herself or letting you do it. Remember that it is her baby, not yours.

Dim the lights. Turn the TV volume off. Make sure the room is warm. These actions create a relaxing atmosphere. Once the baby is skin-to-skin, pull the sheet or blanket over both mother and baby, and pull up a chair for yourself. Sitting at her side communicates your willingness to engage and spend time with her. If you are a staff person, on your feet all day, you relax when you sit, and this will encourage the mother to relax, too.

There is a lot to talk about. Ask her about the birth. Ask if the baby looks like anyone she knows. Go through some of the discharge teaching topics. Ask who will be home to wait on her hand and foot for a week or two, so she can recover from the birth and establish breastfeeding.

In about half the cases, the mother's facial expression will show wonder and surprise as her baby self-attaches under the sheet, with no effort on her part. In the other cases, the baby will sink into deep sleep. Then have the mother hand express, collect her milk on a spoon, and have her feed it to her baby. A sleeping baby can be spoon fed easily. Encourage her to do this whenever she feels her baby should eat. No matter what happens in the room, the mother has had a positive experience.

Skin-to-skin is a personal favorite strategy in breastfeeding rehabilitation. After years of work, it has demonstrated its value beyond any doubt.

Glover and Wiessinger say it well, "Encourage (the mother) to begin as many feeds as possible with skin-to-skin time… encouraging the mother to enjoy ample skin-to-skin time with her baby and to follow her baby's lead are the most important steps of all" (Glover & Wiessinger, 2008).

Massage Techniques for Mother and Baby

Massage techniques have their place in the lactation professional's repertoire as ways to improve the maternal-infant relationship, increase milk supply, increase milk flow, reduce mastitis, and increase infant weight gain.

Regular touch in a daycare center gentled four- and five-year-olds prone to aggressive behavior. Aggressive children were randomized into two groups. The experimental group was massaged at naptime for five to ten minutes once a day; the control group heard a story instead. Over the year of the study period, the massaged children were gentler in daycare and calmer at home. Their parents reported a decrease in somatic complaints. "Daily massage for five to ten minutes could be an easy and cheap way to decrease aggression among preschool children" (von Knorring, Soderberg, Austin, & Uvnas-Moberg, 2008). In another study, massage had a calming effect on aggressive adolescents who received two chair massages weekly for one month (Diego et al., 2002).

Newborn babies touch their mothers with purpose when immediately placed skin-to-skin after birth. Their legs massage her belly as they crawl toward the breast, keeping her womb contracted, so it doesn't bleed. Once they reach her breast, their hands massage it. This hand massage is part of the self-attachment process first documented by Righard and Alade (1990). Crawling to and massaging the mother's breast encourages infant suckling, as the massage releases oxytocin that makes the milk flow. "Periods of increased massage-like hand movements or sucking of the mother's breast were followed by increasing maternal oxytocin levels (p<0.005)" (Matthieson, Ransjo-Arvidson, Nissen, & Uvnas-Moberg, 2001).

Pleasure in touch and in relationship can be measured by oxytocin levels that rise in both the person receiving and in the person giving massage (Uvnäs-Moberg, 2003). In massage, it is as blessed to give as to receive!

Massage Benefits in the Neonatal Intensive Care Nursery

Dr. Tiffany Field documented increased weight gain and earlier discharge of premature infants from the intensive care nursery after they received one 15-minute massage per shift for ten days (Field et al., 1986). The massaged neonates had an average 47% increased weight gain per day when compared with non-massaged infants. Their hospital stay was six days shorter than the control infants. It is interesting to note that no infants in this study were breastfed. They were all bottle-fed infant formula and all received similar amounts of food, yet the massaged infants gained the most weight. Another study by the same author showed a similar improvement with a 15-minute massage once a shift for five days (Dieter, Field, Hernandez-Reif, Emory, & Redzepi, 2003).

One of the most common questions parents ask about their babies in the NICU is, "When can my baby come home?" If infant massage was part of NICU routine care, more babies would go home sooner, families would be reunited, and costs for a hospital stay would decrease.

Babies like the right type of touch. Premature infants prefer massage of moderate firmness (Field, Diego, Hernandez-Reif, Deeds, & Figuereido, 2006). If the touch is too light, it doesn't stimulate as much weight gain.

Massage of premature infants yields other benefits. Massaged babies' bones increase in mineral density when passive range of motion is added to the massage routine (Vignochi, Miura, & Canani, 2008; Moyer-Mileur, Ball, Brunstetter, & Chan, 2008). Massage protects very premature infants from sepsis and gets them home faster than infants receiving standard care (Mendes & Procianoy, 2008).

When intensive care nursery staff massaged premature infants (Yellott, 2001), the parents became receptive to both learning and to using massage techniques with their babies. The massage skills helped parents overcome feelings of inadequacy and promoted a positive relationship with the babies. Dr. Field reports that 38% of 84 neonatologists surveyed reported the use of infant massage in their NICUs (Field, Diego, & Hernandez-Reif, 2010). Research findings are put in practice at the Arnold Palmer NICU in Hollywood, Florida, where there are four infant massage instructors on staff. Dawn Hawthorne, CNM, MS, IBCLC, a clinical director, considers the massage to be one of the life saving elements of the care. (Another is using human milk for all infants; donor milk when mother's own milk is not available.)

Theories About Why Massage Promotes Weight Gain

Currently, there are three theories explaining the connection between infant massage and infant weight gain:

1) Massage stimulates the vagus nerve, thus relaxing organs (Diego, Field, Hernandez-Reif., 2005; Diego et al., 2007). The vagus, the tenth cranial nerve, called the "wanderer" because it makes contact with all internal

organs, has a powerful impact on organ functions. Stimulation of the vagus can reduce pain (Kirchner, Birklein, Stefan, & Handwerker, 2000). Increases in gastric motility as the result of vagal stimulation may contribute to better absorption of nutrients and may explain the weight gain in the premature infant. Vagal stimulation also contributes to an increase in insulin levels, another factor associated with weight gain. Perhaps massage also reduces a premature infant's pain, facilitating weight gain. This is an area for further study.

2) Insulin levels and insulin-like growth factor 1 levels are higher after massage (Field, Diego, et al., 2008). Both insulin and insulin-like growth factor promote growth by increasing the conversion of glucose to lipids and stimulating cell growth. Massage also decreases levels of the stress hormone cortisol, which interferes with the action of insulin. Stress is a barrier to weight gain, as manifested in the stunted growth of the Romanian orphans.

3) Massage reduces metabolic demand, so massaged babies burn fewer calories (Lahat, Mimouni, Ashbel, & Dollberg, 2007). Infant weight gain is also related to the calming effects of massage that reduce infant crying. Since crying is an aerobic activity for an infant, infants that cry for long periods may have problems gaining weight.

Breastfed full-term infants also gain more weight when massaged. Nurses in health centers in Santiago, Chile, taught 35 mothers how to massage their babies, while 65 other mothers were not taught. Mothers in both groups were similar in socioeconomic status and demographic factors. Mothers were encouraged to give one massage a day, starting at two weeks postpartum. At two months postpartum, the babies that had been massaged weighed more than the 65 control group babies. While there were no differences between weights at four months postpartum, the authors concluded that daily massage had a positive impact on the infants' early weight gain. About 5% more mothers were breastfeeding exclusively at two and at four months in the massage group, although the researchers didn't consider this to be a significant difference (Serrano, Doren, & Wilson, 2010). The evidence is strong enough to recommend infant massage when an infant's slow weight gain is of concern.

The evidence is unequivocal that massage is good for babies. It is also good for mothers. Massaged adults have lower blood pressure and pulse rates, and lower levels of cortisol and other stress hormones (Uvnäs-Moberg, 2003). The World Health Organization and UNICEF include a section about maternal massage in their Breastfeeding Counseling Training Course. Session 20 of the Participant's Manual encourages breastfeeding helpers to give a mother a back rub as a way to stimulate oxytocin release.

A description of how to give a back rub is illustrated (Figure 30 in the manual). The helper is taught how to position the mother, where to touch, and to use firm pressure with her thumbs when massaging (WHO, 2011).

Nursing students used to be taught to give back rubs as a way to increase patient comfort, improve circulation, and relieve pain. Nurses working on evening (3:00 PM to 11:00 PM) shift on medical-surgical wards in the 1970s gave a back massage as part of routine bedtime care. Giving a massage to our clients is not part of current lactation education or practice, but it should be. Breastfeeding helpers might consider integrating some basic massage techniques into their work, once the mother understands and gives permission. Massage relaxes a mother and lactation therapist alike, and creates an environment that promotes open discussion.

The Role of Massage in Mother-Baby Communication

Mothers with breastfeeding difficulties may have difficulty understanding or communicating with their infant. They can be mystified by or unable to respond appropriately to infant cues. Some mothers don't respond to infant signals at all. How many of us have witnessed a mother window-shopping, oblivious to her screaming infant in the stroller she is pushing? How many have seen a mother ignoring or not recognizing infant feeding cues, or using a pacifier to keep the baby silent and looking at the clock to regulate feeding? How many mothers interpret their baby's slightest vocalization as "fussiness," which must be soothed or stifled immediately? I have witnessed parents forcibly holding a pacifier in a screaming infant's mouth. These are signs of a disruption in maternal-infant communication. Most babies need far more contact than is culturally sanctioned in the U.S.

For contrast with U.S. baby-tending practices, here is one example of a mother with Kenyan roots, Claire Niala, who writes of her grandmother's advice to her after giving birth to her first baby. "Offer the breast every single moment that baby is upset–even if just fed. Sleep with your baby. Have water nearby at night to keep (you) hydrated. Make the feeding a priority. Read your baby, not the books. Breastfeeding is not linear… you are the expert on your baby's needs" (Niala, 2010). Ms. Niala describes the differences between babies in the U.K. (where infant crying is considered a normal part of life) and babies in Kenya (where a baby crying is cause for alarm and immediate attention; Barr, 1999).

Infants from the U.S., Holland, and the !Kung San in Botswana initiate crying with the same frequency. However, the !Kung San infants sustain crying for more than 30 seconds for less than 10% of crying events in the first nine months of their lives. Why the difference? !Kung San mothers respond to infants' noise immediately; whereas, mothers in the U.S. and Holland delay their response.

Breastfeeding works best when the mother quickly responds to her newborn, learns what it wants, and offers it. There is a belief in the U.S. that responding to an infant "too quickly" will "spoil" the baby (Barr, 1999); this can lead mothers to do anything except breastfeeding or picking the baby up to quiet the baby. Mothers who respond to infant noises by using a plastic device or a gadget (inserting a pacifier or putting a baby in an infant swing or bouncy seat) can benefit by learning that it is effective, pleasurable, fast, and easy to respond with touch and holding and breastfeeding. Infant massage education includes instruction about engaging and responding to the baby, and to stop a particular stroke if the baby becomes distressed.

While responding to infant crying too quickly is viewed as poor parenting because it will "spoil" the baby, infant crying is a source of distress for parents. Many women will wean from breastfeeding if their baby is fussy or crying (Barr, 1999). Daily infant massage is calming (for parent and for baby) and may reduce the risk of premature weaning. Mothers report that massage is easy to integrate into infant care activity, such as diaper change or bathing.

There are several types of infant tummy massage techniques. These techniques have been shown to reduce colic and constipation (Lämås, Lindholm, Stenlund, Engstrom, & Jacobsson, 2009). Lämås et al. concluded that abdominal massage reduced both constipation and laxative use. Mothers (as it is usually mothers that are learning to massage) are taught to stroke in the direction of gut flow, and move their hands or fingers in a clockwise direction on their baby's abdomen. Slow, firm, and loving repetitive stroking can be soothing to both the fussy baby and its parent. When the baby stops the long bouts of crying, the tension level is lowered in the home and everybody feels better.

The Chinese have developed a style of pediatric massage to deal with prolonged crying or colic. Traditional Chinese Medicine has two diagnoses for the baby with colic: Night Crying and/or Abdominal Pain. A child that is relatively calm during the day, but cries either sporadically or continually throughout the night, is manifesting Night Crying. Abdominal Pain is diagnosed by careful observation of the baby's facial expression, leg movements, crying with the back arched backwards, and continuing to cry after a diaper change. The whole framework for diagnosing and treating colic depends on the infant's signs and symptoms, whether they are a spleen vacuity pattern, a fright pattern, a heat bind pattern, a cold pattern, or a food damage pattern. Techniques used to treat each of these patterns are unique and specific (Fan, 2004). Dr. Fan states in her introduction, "The parents' caress is the foundation of the child's health" (Fan, 2004). She goes on to describe the unconscious stroking of the new baby by its mother as playing "a very important role in calming the baby's mind and promoting the circulation of their blood… beneficial both psychologically and physically…" (Fan, 2004).

Massage and Its Impact on Mothering

When a mother becomes attuned to her baby and her baby trusts that she will respond quickly and appropriately, both mother and baby find joy in each other, and breastfeeding is easy and fun. Learning infant massage is a formal way for a mother to become acquainted with her baby's sweet body, thus providing the intimate physical contact that increases oxytocin levels, joy, and pleasure. The structured pattern of infant massage can be a comforting framework for a mother whose interaction with her baby has been governed by books, expert opinions, and the clock. A mother benefits from a framework for security, while she learns to trust spontaneity in her mothering. The mother that cannot yet use breastfeeding to comfort and connect with her baby can achieve those results with regular massage.

A mother who can soothe her baby or relieve colic with massage is a mother whose confidence in her mothering increases. Some of the joy in a new relationship is discovering the types of pleasing touch, and learning what messages are conveyed by the loved one's touch. As mothers may have been disconnected from their babies by hospital practices, they have not yet had a chance to explore their babies. I have worked in many situations where the baby is a week or two old and has not yet been explored by its mother. Although she has bathed, clothed, and changed her baby, she hasn't counted fingers and toes or done any close cuddling. In such cases, the consultation has started with the mother being encouraged to completely undress and inspect her baby. Sometimes mothers need this encouragement on the postpartum unit.

I see the impact of infant massage on maternal-infant relationships regularly when leading infant massage classes at an outpatient breastfeeding center. Two 90-minute classes are given a week apart. The first class is noisy and sometimes chaotic. Babies are fussy. Mothers are awkward and tentative while learning the different massage strokes, and they keep their eye on me to see how to do it right. They pay more attention to the instructor than to their baby.

One week later at the second class, there is an obvious difference between the mothers that have been massaging their babies at home and the ones that haven't. When the practiced mother puts her undressed baby on the blanket and warms some massage oil between her palms, her baby becomes alert and calm, watching the mother's face. The massaged babies reach for and vocalize more with their mothers. The mothers are focused on their baby, holding conversations and paying attention. The two of them have little regard for anyone else in the room. The mothers that haven't practiced during the week are still awkward and tentative in touching their babies.

Impact on Maternal-Infant Attachment

Infant massage improves maternal-infant attachment (Lee, 2006). The change in attachment was documented by improvements in maternal responsiveness scores. The association between infant massage and improved maternal-infant interaction is also observed in studies of mothers with depression, as identified by the Edinburgh Postnatal Depression Scale. The impact of infant massage was found in situations where one group of depressed mothers was assigned to attend both an infant massage class and a support group, while another group was assigned to attend a support group only. Both groups of mothers had a reduction in their EPDS scores, but only the group of mothers in the infant massage class showed an improvement in the mother-infant interaction score (Onozawa, Glover, Adams, Modi, & Kumar, 2001; Field, 2010; O'Higgins, St James Roberts, & Glover, 2008).

A study of mothers of premature infants validates that infant massage improves the maternal-infant relationship (Ferber et al., 2005). In the group where the mothers regularly massaged their premature infants, at three months after hospital discharge, the mothers were less likely to interrupt their babies' activities, their babies were more social, and there was more reciprocity in the relationship when compared with the control infants who did not receive massage.

Other Types of Massage Useful in Lactation

Breast massage is a strategy for increasing milk supply and increasing fat content in milk; useful for a mother collecting milk for a premature infant and for a baby with less than optimal weight gain. Colleagues that have experience with dairy animals have spoken about the benefits of hand expression as a way to physically dislodge fat globules from the walls of the ducts, so they enter the milk. "I remember my uncle saying that hand milking got a better yield than machines" (K. Frantz, personal communication, March 2010). In 1988, Stutte and colleagues published a paper showing that breast massage increased fat content of human milk (Stutte, Bowles, & Morman, 1988).

Alternate breast massage, where the mother massages her breast when the baby pauses between suckles, is reported to increase milk supply and reduces the incidence and severity of engorgement (Walker, 2000). Dr. Jack Newman calls this technique "breast compression." A study from California found that pump-dependent mothers of premature infants increased their mean daily milk volume using breast massage before and during pumping (Morton et al., 2009).

Oketani Massage

Oketani is a specialized form of breast massage practiced in Japan, named after its founder, midwife Sotomi Oketani. The website (www.oketani-school.jp) gives history, describes the courses offered, and encourages midwives to learn the skill. Midwife Kono Okeya formalized a method of breast massage in 1981, as a way to improve infant survival based on the experiences of midwives working in China during World War II. Oketani breast massage is said to improve lactation, soften the breast, and increase the pliability of the areola and nipple, although I could find no studies to support those claims. Practitioners say that the result is an easier milk flow, the quality of the milk improves, and the mother becomes more relaxed. In 2008 there were over 400 Oketani Certified practitioners in Japan, working in hospitals and clinics. Hospitals offer breast massage courses for expectant parents because of its positive relationship with milk supply (Ayers, 2000).

In 2004, Foda and colleagues published a study showing that milk composition changed as a result of Oketani breast massage. Two groups of mothers, one in early lactation (before 90 days postpartum) and the other in late lactation (between 91 and 320 days postpartum) collected milk samples by hand expression before and after breast massage. Analysis of the pre- and post-massage samples revealed an increase in milk solids and gross energy content. Lipid content increased only in the late lactation mothers. Dr. Foda speculates that the changes may be the result of oxytocin and prolactin excretion. He cites a PhD thesis (in Japanese) where the researcher discovered that Oketani breast massage increased the average amount of a small peptide in 11 of 15 mothers, and decreased the lipoxygenase activity in 23 of 27 subjects. The value of this change is not known, although the researcher is quoted by Foda as saying that there may be some antiallergenic effect from Oketani breast massage. Here is another interesting area for research (Foda, Kawashima, Nakamura, Kobayashi, & Oku, 2004).

Breast massage is said to relieve breast pain, relieve lymphatic congestion, reduce pain from lumps or cysts, reduce discomfort during pregnancy, and reduce engorgement during weaning (Massage London, 2011). Some complementary practitioners recommend it as a component of daily health maintenance.

Mammology Practices in Russia

In Russia, physicians known as mammologists specialize in breast massage used therapeutically to relieve the above-mentioned breast conditions. Maya Bolman, RN, BSN, BA, IBCLC, has witnessed first-hand the Russian techniques used by mammologists who work with breastfeeding mothers. Mammologists use specialized techniques to relieve mastitis and engorgement, claiming to do so in one session. I couldn't find any studies about these techniques.

Ms. Bolman visited Russia in September 2009 and taught seminars for local lactation consultants. In turn, they taught her techniques of breast massage and manual expression. Ms. Bolman reports that the Russian experts have developed exquisite skills of manual assessment, and are able to identify exactly where the blockage lies in the breast (called "lactostasis"), then use massage to relieve the block and get the milk to flow. Ms. Bolman is presently compiling all the video clips she made into one, and plans to share this with the lactation community soon.

Lymphatic Drainage Therapy

Lymphatic drainage therapy is a type of subtle massage that works with the physiology of the lymphatic system. Practitioners learn to evaluate the rhythm, direction, depth, and quality of lymph flow, and use specific techniques to improve that flow. Benefits of lymphatic drainage include reduction in edema and relief of pain. Relief from breast engorgement is the major anecdotal finding, as any formal evidence is non-existent. The founder of lymphatic drainage therapy presented the modality at the 1999 ILCA conference (Chikly, 1999), inspiring some conference attendees to learn more about it.

Lactation consultants have reported that lymphatic drainage therapy is useful (Wilson-Clay & Hoover, 2008). Ms. Wilson-Clay referred three clients with pathologic engorgement to receive lymphatic drainage therapy. All three reported that their symptoms were relieved, and they got more milk during pumping after the treatment. There are no reports of any harm done using lymphatic drainage therapy.

Coining (Gua-Sha)

Coining or Gua-Sha, a practice common in Thailand, Vietnam, and China, is a technique whereby the edge of a spoon or a coin is rubbed on the skin. The goal of the technique is to release excess wind. Coining creates a particular skin mark that looks like a red stripe. Sometimes Tiger Balm or some other lubricant is used; the skin is never broken. I am unaware of any formal education in this technique that is currently available to practitioners in the U.S., and advise caution to any breastfeeding helper that would recommend it.

The efficacy of Gua-Sha in the postpartum for a mother with breast fullness is described in a case report; only the abstract is available in English (Chiu, Chang, & Gau, 2008). Gua-Sha was used in addition to giving the mother practical advice and encouragement, ensuring that latch and positioning were accurate, and performing regular follow-up. The goal of the Gua-Sha was to help the milk to flow and to reduce her breast discomfort. The mother continued breastfeeding. From a Western point of view, the Gua-Sha might seem to be the least effective of the four therapeutic strategies; from the mother's and practitioner's points of view, all four were necessary and useful.

A randomized controlled trial of Gua-Sha therapy for breast engorgement compared Gua-Sha with the traditional breast care of massage and heating given to the control group. The Gua-Sha protocol consisted of lightly scraping appropriate acupoint positions. Fifty-four postpartum women with breast engorgement were enrolled. One group received Gua-Sha treatment, the other group received hot packs and 20 minutes of massage. At the start of the study, each group had identical body temperature, breast temperature, engorgement, and levels of discomfort and pain. Five and 30 minutes after the treatment, the groups had statistically different scores ($P<.001$); with the Gua-Sha treatment group showing reduction in engorgement, discomfort, and pain levels. The conclusion and implications for practice are that Gua-Sha therapy can be used to relieve breast engorgement by a skilled practitioner (Chiu et al, 2010).

DiSandro Breast Massage

Diane DiSandro, BA, IBCLC, is a lactation consultant with many years of varied and fascinating clinical experience, and is a sought-after speaker at local conferences. She has developed a unique technique of breast massage that she uses for the treatment of recurrent mastitis. In her own words (and with her permission):

I developed this (technique) when working with a postpartum mom who was starting her third 7- to 10-day course of antibiotics for mastitis; her baby was only six weeks old. This mom wanted to wean, but couldn't even accomplish that without developing mastitis. Nothing was working.

I imagined what would happen if there were a fibroid cyst or some other structural anomaly lying on a milk duct, and repeatedly not allowing it to drain properly. No matter how well we drained and treated it, the problem would just keep happening. Instead of massaging the breast as usual (from outer in towards nipple), I had the mom imagine that her breast was a bag of marbles. She was to pick up the breast and "knead" it, or rather "mush" it around. This is what I would say: "Place the heels of your hands at the outer edge of breast (around 3 and 9 o'clock), with fingertips up slightly interlacing over the nipple. Now, knead IN with your fingertips and also knead with your palms and thumbs. The idea is to move each little marble a millimeter or so to the left or right. Just a slight shift, since we can't really move them far. Do this three to four times per day, in the morning shower, at lunchtime, dinnertime, and at bedtime. Just move those little cysts (or whatever) a little bit, and later, move them somewhere else a bit."

I have used this technique with too many moms to count over the years now. It really works well when everything else has been addressed and the recurrent plugs or mastitis continues.

This creativity in lactation management by pioneers in the field is inspirational! Note that the lactation professional sustains contact with the mother until the problem is resolved.

Reverse Pressure Softening

Another type of gentle massage is called reverse pressure softening (RPS), and works to move fluid away from the nipple and areola, so there is room in a turgid breast for a baby to latch on. A scholarly article in the *Journal of Human Lactation* ascribes three benefits to RPS: it promotes milk ejection reflex, reduces tension on the areas of ductal branching under the areola, and moves edema away from the nipple (Cotterman, 2004). The technique consists of using either fingertips or flats of fingers to press completely around the base of the nipple; the firm and comfortable pressure is maintained for one to three minutes or a slow count of 50.

Areolar Compression

In a lovely case of great minds simultaneously thinking alike, the same issue of the *Journal of Human Lactation* features a case study where a mother was taught to move edema away from her nipple, towards the base of the breast, so that her nipple would become pliable and easily grasped by her nursing baby. The technique used in this study is called Areolar Compression (AC), and is also effective (Miller & Riordan, 2004). Both articles feature lovely close-up views of the techniques and their impact on breast and areola edema. When mothers massaged their breast in this way every two hours, they reported relief of symptoms and improved milk flow 24 hours later.

Speculation about Infant Massage and Breastfeeding

As infant massage of the mother's breast increases oxytocin levels, oxytocin levels increase during massage, and since oxytocin is the hormone of milk flow, maternal massage of the infant should, by extension, improve breastfeeding (Turner, Altemus, Enos, Cooper, & McGuinness, 1999), while supporting the mothering relationship. As massage improves the mother-infant relationship and as contact increases milk volume and flow, it makes sense that teaching a mother to massage her baby is a way to strengthen their fundamental connection and open the door to breastfeeding. Recommend it to mothers who come for help; teach massage techniques to clients. When the dyad starts to have more fun with each other, when they relax together, breastfeeding has a better chance to succeed.

The link between infant massage and improved breastfeeding has not yet been identified in the literature beyond anecdotal reports, although Dr. Tiffany Field, Director of the Touch-Research Institute in Miami, Florida, says, "… positive effects would be expected" (T. Field, personal communication, March 20, 2010). Mothers in my private practice have enjoyed learning some massage techniques or attending an infant massage class.

One can find infant massage instructors through websites. Here are three: www.lovingtouch.com, www.infantmassageusa.org, and www.iaim.ws

(the International Association of Infant Massage). These organizations offer training for anyone to become certified to teach infant massage. Certification usually requires three days of didactic training, lots of reading, homework, a practicum (usually offering and administering an infant massage class series), and a final exam. There is a fee to uphold certification, and continuing education is required.

There are over 80 recognized styles of massage. In this chapter, the focus is on those that are helpful in increasing joy and connection between mother and baby, in increasing milk supply, and in relieving particular breast problems–more tools for the breastfeeding helper's toolbox.

Acupuncture

Acupuncture is a discipline that is at least 5,000 years old that promotes healing by treating the body's energy flow patterns. These patterns, called meridians, have been mapped (Joswick, 2011). Fine needles are used to penetrate the skin to a depth between one-quarter inch and one inch on specific locations on the meridians called acupuncture points. Acupuncture points have more electrical conductivity than other areas of skin; what this implies has been subject to interpretation (Ahn, Wu, Badger, Hammerschlag, & Langevin, 2005).

A variation of acupuncture, called acupressure or shiatsu, uses fingertip pressure instead of needles to treatment points on meridians. Both modalities have been used for thousands of years to treat low milk supply.

Personal Experiences

My first exposure to acupuncture was in 1975, when a fascinating film, *The Other Half of the Sky: A China Memoir*, produced by Shirley MacLaine, was shown in the States after President Nixon resumed diplomatic relations with China. Most memorable was the film clip of a mother having a cesarean section with acupuncture being the only analgesia; the mother was awake and being fed tofu during the surgery!

In the 1980s, someone suggested I use a practitioner of Chinese medicine for treatment of my migraine headaches. This practitioner recommended dietary modification based on the differences in food energies. Foods are classified in Chinese medicine as either yin (cooling, expansive), yang (warming, contractive), or neutral. She made a list of yang foods to avoid (chocolate, red meat, red wine, cheese, eggs) and also advised staying away from physically cold foods. Her advice brought life-long (so far) relief. In this instance, the foods to be avoided are the same foods that allopathic practitioners suggest avoiding, although the fundamental rationale is different. Twenty-two years ago, I used licensed acupuncturists for treatment of infertility; the result was born March 26, 1990. My bias in favor of acupuncture is hereby disclosed; success breeds trust.

When this second baby was four years old, a raft of annoying symptoms (insomnia, menstrual flooding and irregularity, vaginal dryness, low energy, and severe hair loss) led me to a Chinese (born, trained, and licensed in China) physician, who spoke little at our first visit. She felt my pulses. She said, "Let me see your tongue." She asked me about my births, "Natural?" "Yes," I replied, proudly remembering two unmedicated spontaneous labors. She looked disappointed and asked, "No bleeding?" Only then did I remember the 1500 cc of blood loss after delivery, four years previous. This hemorrhage had led to the development of sub-clinical hypothyroidism (Razvi, Ingoe, McMillan, & Weaver, 2005). How amazing that she diagnosed this after a touch on my wrist, a glance at my tongue, and two questions. She treated me with acupuncture and herbs; all the symptoms disappeared after four visits, never to return.

Evidence about Acupuncture and Acupressure

Acupuncture has been reviewed by the Cochrane Collaborative and found to be helpful in the treatment of many conditions, including management of labor pain. Acupressure, where the treatment points are pressed instead of needled, was found to be effective in relieving symptoms of hyperemesis gravidarium (Shin, Song, & Seo, 2007). In a randomized control group pretest-posttest design, 66 hospitalized pregnant women were assigned to one of three groups: control (receiving the usual intravenous therapy), placebo (where pressure was applied close, but not directly on the pressure point), and treatment. Improvement in the experimental group was greater than in the other groups, and the difference was statistically significant.

The National Institutes of Health (NIH) said in 1997, "A consensus panel convened by the National Institutes of Health today concluded there is clear evidence that needle acupuncture treatment is effective for postoperative and chemotherapy nausea and vomiting, nausea of pregnancy, and postoperative dental pain…there are a number of other… conditions for which acupuncture may be effective as an adjunct therapy, an acceptable alternative, or as part of a comprehensive treatment program, but for which there is less convincing scientific data. These conditions include, but are not limited to addiction, stroke rehabilitation, headache, menstrual cramps, tennis elbow, fibromyalgia (general muscle pain), low back pain, carpal tunnel syndrome, and asthma" (NIH, 1997). Of particular interest is their statement that "adverse side effects are low, and often lower than conventional (i.e., allopathic) treatments."

The National Institutes of Health reinforced that acupuncture is effective for postoperative pain, chemotherapy-induced nausea and vomiting, and nausea associated with pregnancy (Ayers, 2000). The NIH explains the effectiveness of this Eastern medicine using a Western scientific framework. Perhaps the acupuncture points stimulate blood flow to vital organs or stimulate the release of other neuropeptides that have a therapeutic impact (Mayer, 2000).

In 2008 (Schnyer et al., 2008), the Society for Acupuncture Research elaborated on the value of acupuncture for a wide range of conditions: pain, neurologic conditions, women's health, psychiatric disorders, cancer care, and functional bowel disorders. Their conclusion is that the future holds great promise for selection and utilization of the best of eastern and western medical practices together, an integrative approach.

Ear acupressure is a variation of acupuncture and is a recognized modality in European folk medicine (Gori & Firenzuoli, 2007). The Ebers Papyrus from 1550 B.C. contains a description of channels in the body that approximates more closely the Chinese system of channels than any other written organization of blood or lymph vessels or nerves. Women in ancient Egypt had their ear pricked with a needle or cauterized for contraception. Hippocrates said that doctors of the time opened veins behind the ear to treat impotency and facilitate ejaculation. Physicians in the 17th, 18th, and 19th centuries in Europe told of various treatments given to the external ear to treat sciatica, toothache, and leg pain. Dr. Paul Nogier, a French physician, observed in the 1950s that specific points on the ear, when stimulated, would have an impact on specific body organs. He is considered to be the father of modern auricolotherapy. Dr. Nogier made a famous drawing of the inverted fetus overlaid over a drawing of the external ear to illustrate how points on the ear represent body structures (Gori & Firenzuoli, 2007).

Ear acupuncture was analgesic for 90 patients with cancer pain. Pain intensity decreased by 36% in the group receiving auricular acupuncture, but only 2% in those patients in the control group (p< 0.0001; Alimi et al., 2003).

Acupuncture and Acupressure in Breastfeeding Rehabilitation

The Chinese scientific literature shows that acupuncture is effective in increasing milk supply and infant weight gain. "Other things being equal, infants whose mothers received Traditional Chinese Acupuncture (TCA) weighed 160.13 grams more on average than infants whose mothers received Sham Acupuncture" (Li, 2003). While this particular study is limited by both a small number of subjects and a low participation rate, it does open the door to further research. Another study (Clavey, 1996) recommends stimulation of the point identified as 'small intestine 1' and specific points on the areola when done five to seven days postpartum, as an effective way to increase milk supply.

In the case of a 41-year-old woman receiving acupuncture for the relief of pain after a mastectomy who then developed galactorrhea, the report states that, "…there is quantitative evidence that acupuncture… causes the release of prolactin and oxytocin." The subject had weaned four years earlier; CT and MRI scans of her brain showed no abnormality (Jenner & Filshie, 2002). Other research concludes that acupuncture increases prolactin and oxytocin levels. Chinese science says that insufficient milk supply may be the result of either a spleen chi deficiency or a liver stagnation. If the spleen energy is lacking, milk production is inadequate. If the liver energy is stagnant, the breasts are full, but the milk doesn't flow (Li, 2003).

Swedish midwives found that mastitis symptom severity indices (measuring breast tension, redness, and pain) were significantly different between the group receiving acupuncture and the group that didn't (Kvist, Hall-Lord, Rydhstroem, & Larsson, 2007). Their conclusion is that acupuncture, if acceptable to the mother, could be a useful adjunct to the standard measures for lactational breast inflammation and that it may relieve engorgement or inflammation enough that milk can flow.

The Cochrane Review about treatment for breast engorgement determined that acupuncture made a significant improvement to engorgement symptoms (Mangesi & Dowswell, 2011). Lactation consultants Diana West and Lisa Marasco are internationally renowned experts in the treatment of low milk supply; they include a page on acupuncture and acupressure as useful modalities on their website.[27]

At the 2003 International Conference on the Theory and Practice of Human Lactation Research and Breastfeeding Management, Drs. Hong Yun and Danyun Lu, from China, gave a clinical skill-building presentation about increasing milk supply through ear acupressure. They described the ear as a microcosm of the body as a whole; any disorder of the body may be treated with needling or acupressure at specific points on the external ear. They cited a 4,000-year-old text, the *Jeijing of Inner Canon of the Yellow Emperor*, that identified specific acupuncture points on the external auricle to use in treatment of low milk supply. These specific ear points enervate and stimulate the liver, stomach, spleen, and endocrine organs.

A participant at the conference, struggling for months with low milk supply, offered to be a subject. Her milk volume increased measurably between the day the treatment was done and the end of the conference two days later. One case study is the lowest level of evidence; success could have

27   http://www.lowmilksupply.org/acupunctureandacupressure.shtml#3

come from the placebo effect, from the attention generated in a public experiment, or by the impact of wearing a newly designed breast pump for many hours a day. Nevertheless, it was impressive to witness.

A recent Chinese study observed that more women in the group treated at acupuncture point Tuina had sufficient lactation, higher prolactin levels, and quicker time to lactation than controls. All mothers in both groups received instruction in and evaluation of breastfeeding. While the prolactin levels were significantly different between the two groups (28 women each), there are still too many questions about this study to support its validity. How was "sufficient lactation" defined? What day postpartum were the women? How was "time to start to lactate" defined and determined? What was the instruction? Unfortunately, only the abstract is available; however, the finding does align itself with positive results from other studies (Lu, Qiu, Yao, & Zheng, 2010).

Finding a Practitioner

Acupuncture is a valuable modality, and one that can be helpful in breastfeeding management. Word of mouth in one's community is a good way to find a safe and reliable acupuncturist. Another way is to use the Internet to find a credentialed practitioner. There are many sets of initials signifying a practitioner who uses acupuncture; these range from ABT (Asian Bodywork Therapist) to TCMD (Traditional Chinese Medicine Doctor).[28]

Regulations for licensure vary from state to state. Some insurance programs pay for acupuncture.

China is a country with a population that is about one-sixth of the world's total. As the Chinese have been using acupuncture and acupressure for at least 5,000 years, we can trust that acupuncture and acupressure have had enough success for enough clients to include it in the lactation toolbox. Consider it for cases of low milk supply, engorgement, lingering aches and pains of delivery, insomnia, and mastitis.

---

28   http://www.acupuncturetoday.com/abc/titlesandabbreviations.php

Chiropractic

Chiropractic is a hands-on modality that can be of marvelous assistance to breastfeeding recovery. When the musculoskeletal system of the mother or the baby has been injured through labor and delivery, breastfeeding can suffer. A gentle and skilled chiropractor can promote healing by treating the musculoskeletal system in mother and in baby.

Chiropractic is defined by The American Chiropractic Association as a healthcare profession that focuses on disorders of the musculoskeletal and nervous systems, primarily the spine, and seeks to restore the healthy relationship between the body's structure and its function. Doctors of Chiropractic practice a drug-free, hands-on approach that includes patient examination, assessment, diagnosis, and treatment. Chiropractors have broad diagnostic skills; they can recommend therapeutic and rehabilitative exercises, as well as provide nutritional, dietary, and lifestyle counseling.

History

Dr. David Palmer formally organized modern chiropractic medicine in 1895. However, spinal adjustment techniques have been described in medical documents for thousands of years. A Chinese document from 2700 B.C. refers to the use of spinal manipulation. Hippocrates wrote about spinal manipulation in two books, discussing diagnosis and using manipulation to treat luxations (the dislocation of a joint) and subluxations (a partial dislocation of a joint). He described using directed pressure to treat scoliosis. During the Middle Ages, Hippocrates' writings were discovered by scholars and used by practitioners in Europe and the Middle East. In the sixteenth century, Ambrose Paré taught and used the manipulation techniques described by Hippocrates. In the eighteenth century, laypeople called 'bonesetters' treated people using spinal manipulation. By the end of the eighteenth century, physicians routinely used manipulation. By the end of the nineteenth century, spinal manipulation was considered risky and had faded from medical practice until it was revived by the Drs. Palmer (father Daniel and son Bartlett).

Concepts and Practice

The signature therapeutic procedure performed by doctors of chiropractic is called an adjustment. Its purpose is to restore joint mobility by manually applying a controlled force into joints that have become restricted in their movement, misaligned, or dislocated. The major focus of chiropractic adjustments is the spine. Restrictions and misalignments can be caused by a single traumatic event, such as improper lifting of a heavy object, an automobile or sports accident, a difficult birth, or through prolonged repetitive movement. Whatever the cause, joints, particularly of the spine, can be affected, causing inflammation, pain, and diminished function. Swelling can impinge onto other body structures, such as nerves and blood or lymph vessels. Manipulation, or adjustment of the affected joint and tissues, moves the joint into optimal physiologic alignment, thereby restoring mobility, alleviating pain and muscle tightness, releasing impingement on other tissues, and enabling the body to heal itself. The controlled force used in manipulation, from light fingertip to directed high velocity touch, varies with the style of chiropractic.

A Doctor of Chiropractic, D.C., has completed a four-year post-baccalaureate program and passed a state licensing examination. There are six different styles of chiropractic: Network Chiropractic, Network Spinal Analysis, Applied Kinesiology, Objective Straight, Mixer, Reform, and Palmer/Straight (the oldest form). All have different philosophies, yet are similar in that their work involves the laying-on of hands.

A chiropractor will evaluate the symmetry and range of motion of all the muscles, bones, and joints of the mother and the baby. Sometimes the chiropractor will give the parents exercises to do with the baby to relax particular muscles and help bones achieve proper alignment.

The Difference Between a Chiropractor and an Osteopath

The difference between chiropractic and osteopathy is not always easily determined. In the 21st century, there is little left that is as pure as it was before radio, TV, easy international travel, and the Internet. When new information is brought to awareness, practitioners are changed. There are now more forms of Chiropractic than there were 150 years ago, as concepts of energy medicine, nutrition, and other disciplines have been adopted, transforming the original practice into modern variations.

Osteopaths today function like allopathic physicians; they perform surgery, treat acute medical illness, and write medical prescriptions. While osteopaths are taught spinal manipulation, the newer, younger practitioners use it rarely. I worked as a nurse in maternity at an osteopathic hospital in the 1990s. The resident osteopaths practiced obstetrics in a way that was indistinguishable from that of the medical obstetricians. The only difference was that the osteopaths would write an order for spinal manipulation to the lumbar spine to be done three times a day, although I never saw it performed by any, but one (older) practitioner.

Osteopathy is also useful in breastfeeding rehabilitation. A recent case report describes the osteopathic treatment given to premature twins who were unable to take enough nutrition via nipple, and gastrostomy tube placement was planned. The osteopathic treatments (including myofascial release, inhibition pressure, cranial decompression, and hyoid bone balancing) resolved their structural difficulties, so they were able to progress to full oral feeds and avoid gastrostomy tubes (Lund et al., 2011). If there is a good osteopath in your community, include them in your referral network of specialists.

Unlike osteopaths, chiropractors do not attend patients in hospitals, write medical prescriptions, or perform surgery. They do not treat acute medical illness.

Insurance will reimburse both osteopathy and chiropractic, depending on the individual's plan. The U.S. Department of Health and Human Services says that conventional medicine is practiced by holders of MD (medical doctor) or DO (doctor of osteopathy) degrees (NCCAM, 2009).

History of the Mistrust Between Allopathy and Chiropractic

Some medical doctors are resistant to and skeptical about chiropractic. This attitude has historical roots, which led to years of legal action from 1976 to 1987.

The American Medical Association's Principles of Medical Ethics held that it was unethical for medical doctors to associate with "unscientific practitioners" and labeled chiropractic "an unscientific cult." In 1958, the AMA's Section 3 of Principles of Medical Ethics stated: "A physician should practice a method of healing founded on a scientific basis; and he should not voluntarily associate professionally with anyone who violates this principle" (American Medical Association, 1957). In 1963, the AMA formed a Committee on Quackery, whose express purpose was to eliminate chiropractic from the healthcare professions (Whitelaw, 2002). This committee was disbanded in 1974.

Chester A. Wilk, DC, was one of four chiropractors to initiate an antitrust suit against the AMA in 1976.[29] In 1987, the U.S. District Court ruled that the AMA was guilty of conspiracy in restraint of trade, a violation of the Sherman Act (Chiropractic Resource Organization, 2010, p. 46). The AMA lost its appeal to the U.S. Court of Appeals; the Supreme Court refused to hear the case at all. The AMA from that time forward has had to allow its members to collaborate with DCs.

Presiding District Court Judge Susan Getzendanner said, "Evidence at the trial showed that the defendants took active steps… to undermine chiropractic educational institutions, conceal evidence of the usefulness of chiropractic care, undercut insurance programs for patients of chiropractors, subvert government inquiries into the efficacy of chiropractic, engage in a massive disinformation campaign to discredit and destabilize the chiropractic profession, and engage in numerous other activities to maintain a medical physician monopoly over healthcare in this country." Judge Getzendanner also stated, "I decline to pronounce chiropractic valid or invalid on anecdotal evidence, even though the anecdotal evidence in the record favors chiropractors" (Chiropractic Resource Organization, 2010).

This legal action had positive outcomes. One is that the AMA abolished Principle 3 and stated that physicians were free to choose with whom to associate and to refer. Another is that chiropractic built a scientific foundation. Chiropractic research is published, and randomized controlled clinical trials support the value of the modality. Today, there are peer-reviewed journals that publish research about chiropractic. PubMed lists the *Journal of Manipulative and Physiologic Therapeutics*, *Journal of the Canadian Chiropractic Association*, and *Chiropractic and Osteopathic Medicine*. Chiropractic research is also published in other peer-reviewed journals, such as *Archives of Disease of Children*.

In 1992, the AMA issued this statement: "It is ethical for a physician to associate professionally with chiropractors provided that the physician believes that such association is in the best interests of his or her patient. A physician may refer a patient for diagnostic or therapeutic services to a chiropractor permitted by law to furnish such services whenever the physician believes that this may benefit his or her patient. Physicians may also ethically teach in recognized schools of chiropractic" (American Medical Association, 1992).

The National Center of Complementary and Alternative Medicine (NCCAM), a division of the National Institutes of Health, has links to overviews, research, and references about chiropractic on their website (NCCAM, 2010). The NCCAM states that spinal manipulation can

29   http://www.chiro.org/Wilk/

provide low to moderate relief for low-back pain. Chiropractic techniques include spinal manipulation and can provide low to moderate relief for this common ailment that affects as many as one-fourth of the adult population (NCCAM, 2009). Current research shows that many people have relief of low-back pain for up to 18 months after treatment. The risk of serious complications is very low when spinal manipulation is performed by a trained and licensed practitioner.

Breastfeeding and Chiropractic

Some babies have injuries at birth that can lead to breastfeeding difficulties or compromised milk supply. Babies can have stiff necks or tilted jaws that interfere with a symmetrical, deep latch. Specific breastfeeding problems that can be relieved by chiropractic are those where the baby latches on poorly, injuring the mother and transferring little milk; when the baby wants to suck every minute all day and night long; can nurse only in one position; or is unable to coordinate suck, swallow, and breathe.

There are anecdotal reports of mothers with milk-making problems who improve when they themselves get chiropractic adjustments. Intercostal nerves 3, 4, and 5 must be working without impediment for signals to travel from the baby's mouth through the nipple to the spinal cord and thence to the pituitary. Anything impinging on those nerves will interfere with their function; chiropractic adjustment reduces interference with nerves.

La Leche League (Vallone, 2004) identifies chiropractic as an effective modality for babies who are injured by vacuum or forceps, whose muscles and bones are not working well together so the baby is in pain, or who are poor feeders. While chiropractic has proved useful in breastfeeding recovery for many according to stories from both lactation professionals and from mothers, published evidence is both scanty and growing.

A case series of 114 babies evaluated the impact of manipulation on babies referred for chiropractic by a medical practitioner for evaluation and treatment of sub-optimal sucking. The definition of sub-optimal infant breastfeeding used in the study was if the infant could not be exclusively fed at breast. Suck was classified according to a suck reflex grading scale developed by the primary author. The biomedical problems diagnosed in the babies were altered tongue action, decreased mandible excursion, hypotonic suprahyoid muscle, displaced hyoid, aberrant cervical range of motion and/or posterior joint restrictions, hypo or hypertonic function of particular muscles (obicularis oris, masseter, digastrics) , and temporomandibular joint laxity or imbalance (Miller, Miller, Sulesund, &

Yevtushenko, 2009). The problems were manifested in an infant's inability to open its mouth wide enough, in its tongue or lips not coordinating with sufficient strength to grasp the breast, or in disturbances of infant posture, balance, and neural function.

The average number of treatment visits was four; the mother monitored improvement. The outcome measure of the study was exclusive breastfeeding. After an average of four treatments, 89 infants (78%) were exclusively breastfeeding. All babies treated showed some improvement. The authors noted that there was a higher than average rate of birth interventions in the cohort.

Parents seek chiropractic care for relief of infantile colic. In one study, 100 infants were randomly assigned to one of two groups. Colic was defined in this study as three hours of crying per day for more than three days per week for the previous three weeks. One group received treatment with spinal manipulation and the other didn't. Eighty-six infants finished the trial. A nurse held the group that did not receive treatment for ten minutes. All the infants were partially undressed. The researchers didn't consider the differences between the groups to be significant; however, more babies in the treated group (69% or 32 of 46) showed improvement in colic symptoms than babies in the untreated group (60% or 24 of 40). There was no evidence of harm (Olafsdottir, Forshei, Fluge, & Markestad, 2001). As colic is attributed to many different causes and a cure for colic has not been discovered, chiropractic is a strategy to consider for some babies.

I have referred dyads to a local chiropractor for relief of the infant's abdominal distress. In one case, the chiropractor used applied kinesiology, a newer technique, to determine the source of the infant's allergies. The baby was treated and showed some relief; however, as his mother was making a number of changes to her diet and receiving craniosacral therapy at the same time as the chiropractic evaluation, it is difficult to associate the improvement with any one modality.

Applied kinesiology uses muscle testing as the primary evaluation method of diagnosis and treatment and may be helpful in the treatment of mastalgia (Gregory, Mills, Hamed, & Fentiman, 2001). When used in allergy testing, one research conclusion was that applied kinesiology may, due to its high sensitivity, be useful in obtaining preliminary results. This same study found moderately high test-retest reliability for the technique (Pothmann, von Frankenberg, Hoicke, Weingarten, & Ludtke, 2001); although, another German study published in the same year concluded that the use of applied kinesiology was no better than guessing (Ludtke, Kunz, Seeber, & Ring, 2001). A more recent review article concludes, "There have been no studies supporting the use of these techniques, and several have refuted their utility. A beneficial placebo effect may be responsible for the perceived clinical effectiveness in many cases of food intolerance" (Teuber & Porch-Curren, 2003). If it is only a beneficial placebo effect, where is the harm, particularly if the situation has improved?

Studies support the use of applied kinesiology. One study of 32 patients from Austria found both therapy localization (another name for applied kinesiology) and homeopathy useful in the treatment of thyroid-associated orbitopathy (Moncayo, Moncayo, Ulmer, & Kainz, 2004).

I find conclusions refuting the use of applied kinesiology disturbing because of personal positive experiences. My daughter, who was taking 180 mg of prescription Allegra™ and steroid nasal spray daily at age 11, stopped using both medications after receiving applied kinesiology from a chiropractor as part of allergy elimination treatments. She has never needed those medicines since then, ten years ago. She has lived in the same house and environment all of her life. Her father stopped snoring after he received applied kinesiology as part of allergy elimination treatments from a chiropractor. No one was expecting (or even hoping) to have his snoring go away; he merely wanted relief from hay fever. My family's experience is not unique.

As has been mentioned before, the breastfeeding helper should know who is available in the community. Word of mouth is an excellent way to find a good local practitioner. There are many complementary and alternative therapies; each has strengths and weaknesses. Each is only as good as the practitioner giving the therapy. Suggest the mother try the practitioner for three visits. If, by the end of that time, there is no improvement, then seek assistance somewhere else.

Many lactation professionals are fortunate to have worked with practitioners that have educated as much as they have treated. Professional dialogue between disciplines is a gift for all.

Craniosacral Therapy

I first heard about craniosacral therapy (CST) in the 1990s from Kay Hoover, M.Ed., IBCLC, FILCA, who recommended it as a technique to resolve persistent breastfeeding difficulties; i.e., situations where, despite intensive lactation management, breastfeeding had not become easy and fun. Trusting her years of experience and her wisdom, I recommended CST to clients with challenges that my lactation management had not resolved, such as the baby clenching while suckling. At that time, paying for lactation services was a novel, and not always welcomed, idea. If lactation services weren't effective, breastfeeding was usually abandoned. Mothers preferred to wean than to spend more money for yet another relatively unknown therapy. After receiving CST treatment myself, thus becoming more convinced of its value, I began studies with the Upledger Institute in 1997 and started blending CST into my clinical practice.

CST is outstanding for its gentleness. It is a non-invasive, hands-on modality. CST aids in breastfeeding recovery by enabling the dyad to recover their connection with each other. It releases tension at a cellular level, altering physical structures.

Sometimes the beneficial effects are so subtle that people deny them. (This also occurs after homeopathic work.) Folks say, "Oh I just happened to sleep well last night" after a treatment and make no connection between treatment and immediate restorative sleep. This is a frustration for a new practitioner. Why would someone deny the connection between lying on my table yesterday and sleeping well that night? They do, despite discussion. My advice is to let it go, and do your best with each person you meet.

CST blends physical with energetic techniques to restore ease and joy to the two people to whom it belongs. There are good feelings and attraction in relationship. Without these, the relationship is joyless and distant. Hospitals rarely remember that the maternity unit is the place where the mother and baby meet for the first time and need to fall in love with each other. Falling in love has nothing to do with feeding method, although love does make breastfeeding easier. I have found CST to remove barriers to the relationship between mother and baby, as well as improving breastfeeding.

What Is Craniosacral Therapy?

Craniosacral therapy is a gentle, non-invasive, hands-on technique used to detect and correct imbalances in the craniosacral system, a scientific approach to the laying on of hands. The body's craniosacral system is made up of the meninges, brain, cerebrospinal fluid, spinal cord, and associated tissues (bone and fascia). The cerebrospinal fluid circulates within the craniosacral system, and bathes and protects the brain and spinal cord.

Human bodies are full of rhythms. Some follow the movement of the earth around the sun, the circadian rhythm; some are energetic, like the afternoon nap, the siesta common in Mediterranean countries, and the increased activity of newborns at night. Hormones and electrolytes peak and ebb in the body in their own rhythms. Nursing mothers are aware of increased breast fullness in the morning, as prolactin levels are higher during the night. Circadian rhythms have been found in human milk components, with fat content changing throughout the day (Lubetsky, Littner, Mimouni, Dollberg, & Mandel, 2006). There are rhythms in the fluids and air driven by our heart and lungs. Cerebrospinal fluid is another fluid whose circulation has a pulse. One can learn to evaluate this pulse, just as one can learn to assess the pulses that reflect organ function in Chinese medicine and just as a physician learns to recognize the many subtleties of cardiac or lung sounds.

The characteristics of the craniosacral rhythm are its symmetry, quality, amplitude, and rate. These are evaluated for diagnosis and treatment. The imbalances and restrictions to the craniosacral rhythm are connected to sensory, motor, or mental dysfunction in the whole body. The CST practitioner evaluates the craniosacral rhythm to learn about the body, to test the significance of various elements to that body, to do some of the techniques that are in the CST repertoire, and to evaluate the impact of the techniques.

The craniosacral system is the core body system. My logo is an illustration of this system:

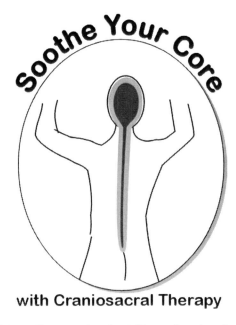

with Craniosacral Therapy

(Thanks to Nancy Zatzman, friend, neighbor and mother of one, for transforming ideas and a sketch into my logo.)

Impact of Birth on the Craniosacral System

A newborn's skull is soft and malleable to fit through the pelvis during birth, and to grow along with its developing brain. The power of birth that spreads the joints of the mother's bones also molds the baby's soft skull. When external force (e.g., from forceps or vacuum or strong hands) is added to the natural pushing forces, there is more pressure and stress on the baby's skull. The shape of the skull is changed, and this changes the shape of the organs inside the skull (brain, spinal cord, and cranial nerves). When the bones change shape, tiny opening in the bones (foramena), where blood vessels and nerves run through, have their shapes distorted. When the foramena's shapes are distorted, the cranial nerves that run through it from the brain to the baby's muscles can be impinged or irritated (Smith, 2010).

The cranial nerves most affecting breastfeeding are the hypoglossal nerve, the pharyngeal nerve, and the vagus nerve, although all are necessary. When these nerves are irritated or constricted, they respond by becoming inflamed, cellular anger that is a response to irritation. There is accompanying alteration of sensory and motor functions in the target organs enervated by those nerves. Alternation in nerve function can lead to a colicky baby, to a muscle that is in spasm, or to a baby with sensory or motor deficits of its mouth and tongue. Altered sensory and motor function can have an impact on breastfeeding and milk removal.

Some cranial molding is helpful, part of the natural process that has been successful for millennia. Exaggerated molding is not helpful; the pulling forces of metal forceps and silicon vacuum cups augment expulsive and molding forces and can damage tissues. As a labor and delivery room nurse, I have seen obstetricians brace their foot on the delivery table in order to pull harder on the baby's head with a vacuum extractor or forceps. Sometimes the pulling, even during a cesarean section, is so strong that the mother is moved down the table.

Caution When Using CST

Upledger Institute training teaches that a person with a fresh head injury, a new stroke, or any situation where the meninges have been punctured (whether it be by spinal tap or by accident), or where blood or cerebrospinal fluid is leaking, should wait for medical clearance before any therapy is used that changes the fluid dynamics of the craniosacral system. If a mother was suffering spinal headaches as a consequence of epidural analgesia, CST would not be recommended until it is certain her meninges are healed. A fluid system must be sealed for therapeutic pressure to do its job.

When the practitioner holds the intention for the greatest good and uses the lightest touch with complete attention on the client, CST will be useful in all other clinical situations.

Intention

The intention of the practitioner has a role in the outcome of any therapy. Intention is what is in our hearts when we act. An example of intention in action is driving to the store–what you most likely do is think, "I am going to the store," and then get into the car and drive there. You don't think, "I have to make a left out of the driveway, go 100 yards, then make a right turn on Cedar Road, and go to the light, and then… etc., etc." Your desire, your reason and motivation to get into the car was to go to the store. Once your intention is set, "go to the store," you drive there.

Imagine putting your hand on someone's arm. What is your intention behind the act? Are you putting your hand on the arm to massage, to evaluate, or to punish? Are you doing it to provide comfort, to restrain, or to stabilize? Are you tickling or teasing or guiding? Are you caressing? While the mechanics of putting a hand on an arm are similar in each of the above situations, the intention of the person wielding the hand determines how the owner of the arm perceives the touch. Best is for the receiving arm to perceive the touch in the way the touching hand intends.

Intention guides our choice of words, and our execution of techniques. Dr. Upledger teaches that when the intention of the therapist and that of the client is congruent, the efficacy of the session is intensified. I ask the mother about her intention behind seeking CST by asking her, "If you had a magic wand, what would you wish for?" or "What would good breastfeeding look like to you?" If she wants to have pain-free breastfeeding, then that thought is in my heart when my hands are on her, and guides my choice of words in dialogue.

Our intention flavors the words we speak and the care we administer. Is it our intention to answer a question quickly because we are busy, have two new admissions, and the end of shift is approaching or is it to encourage dialogue and create an environment where a mother can take the time she needs to express herself? What is the intention of an obstetrician who puts a foot up on the delivery table to brace against while pulling a baby out of a mother by its head using forceps? Is it to provide a respectful, welcoming entrance to this world or is it to get that baby out no matter what? In such situations, the physician's intention has an impact on the mother and the baby, who perceive that intention; breastfeeding can thereby be affected.

Dr. Suzanne Colson writes about intention in her book and asks an important question, "Can the beliefs and attitudes of the health professionals affect breastfeeding outcomes?" (Colson, 2010). Absolutely! The beliefs and attitudes of the practitioners and hospital staff do have an impact on outcome. Think about the intention behind some recommendations given to new mothers. "Don't let your baby use you as a pacifier." "Don't carry your baby in your arms." "Put your baby on a schedule." Will a mother receiving such advice feel comfortable and secure, or will she feel worried about doing something wrong?

A mother came to me after struggling with breastfeeding and fighting with her baby for two months. During a long CST session, she was able to mourn the loss of breastfeeding, stop struggling to make it work, and wholeheartedly accept exclusive pumping. She had lain on the table hoping for a magic event to create the easy breastfeeding she had experienced with her other children. Once deeply relaxed after experiencing several still points (a CST technique whereby the CST rhythm stops and reorganizes, much like a sigh reorganizes breathing and releases tension), she realized that she was unable to do what was necessary to breastfeed this particular baby. The things that had worked with her other four children hadn't worked with this newest baby. She had no time or space for the intensive focus required for breastfeeding rehabilitation (such as spending time every day skin-to-skin with her baby), as she was homeschooling all the other children and because she was a single mother, with an inadequate support network. Letting go of the struggle could occur only when the feelings around her situation were felt, identified, and released; this was the result of a CST session.

History of Craniosacral Therapy

Andrew Taylor Still, M.D., a surgeon during the War Between the States, questioned the medical treatments of his era, which proved futile to save his own children's lives after they contracted meningitis. In the late 1800s, treatment for meningitis included the use of mustard plasters, purging with saline or citrate of magnesia, opium, and shaving the head and applying ice.[30] Dr. Still became particularly skeptical of medications because of their toxic side effects. Grief, curiosity, and keen intellect led to his life-long investigation of the body and of healing. His discoveries led to the development of osteopathy, a new system of medical practice based on four significant healing principles:

1) All body systems are connected. (Today, it is well accepted that the mind, body, and spirit are connected. There is a medical specialty centered on this connection called psychoneuroimmunology.)

2) The site of the presenting pain may not be the origin of the problem. (Allopathic medicine calls this "referred pain.")

3) The body has a self-correcting ability, an inner wisdom, and a drive toward wholeness and healing. Consider a cut on your finger; the Band-Aid doesn't heal the wound. It merely protects it and keeps it clean. The cut heals as a result of the body's self-correcting ability.

4) Body structure and function are related.

Dr. Still is in good company with his attitudes about drugs. Sir William Osler, M.D., the Canadian physician credited with being the father of modern medicine, said, "One of the first duties of the physician is to educate the masses not to take medicine" (Osler, 1860). Oliver Wendell

---

30   http://www.doctortreatments.com/DISEASES-OF-THE-NERVOUS-SYSTEM.html

Holmes, Sr., one-time dean of Harvard Medical School, said in 1860, "… and I firmly believe that if the whole materia medica [medical drugs], *as now used*, could be sunk to the bottom of the sea, it would be all the better for mankind—and all the worse for the fishes" (Osler, 1860).

John Upledger, D.O., is credited with the formalization of craniosacral therapy, using osteopathic principles as a foundation. In his book, *The Inner Physician and You*, he recounts the pivotal case where he was assisting a neurosurgeon during a procedure to remove some debris from a patient's dural tube, the outermost membrane covering the spinal cord. His job was to hold the membrane steady, so the neurosurgeon could scrape off the debris. Dr. Upledger was unable to hold the dural tube still because it had a rhythmic movement. No one had noticed such a phenomenon before (Upledger, 1997).

Craniosacral therapy grew out of Dr. Upledger's curiosity, his interest and skill in other healing modalities, and his foundation in osteopathy. CST is a blending of healing principles from other disciplines that Dr. Upledger found useful. He used the acupuncture concept of meridians, pathways of energy flow that were mapped out in Chinese medicine over 5,000 years ago. From the Vedas, the sacred writings of the Hindu religion that were codified between 600 and 300 B.C., he integrated the assessment and treatment of the chakras.

A CST Session Overview

The clothed mother lies on the table in my quiet and peaceful office. There may be gentle music in the background; the air smells of patchouli or sandalwood, my favorites. The light is natural or from a beeswax candle. The room is quiet; its atmosphere, a sanctuary.

The baby, clad only in a diaper, is lying on her bare chest. Her shoulders may be covered. (This strategy comes from the work of Christina Smillie MD, IBCLC, who has said that a woman will feel more comfortable with exposed breasts if her shoulders are covered.) The mother may need a cover over her body or pillows under her arms; these are provided. The dyad is warm and comfortable.

CST starts at the mother's feet, seeking to ground her to the earth. Seated, with my hands resting lightly on the tops of her feet, it is easy for me to either talk or keep silent while working, as we three settle into a comfortable relationship.

I start at the foot of the table, saying a silent prayer of thanks for this client, wondering what we will learn together, and offering myself to be used for the greatest good. Once I place my hands lightly on her body, my palms can feel like they are melting into the client's skin. I pay attention to the sensations coming to me through my hands.

While adults lie on the table, children may be anywhere. I've worked on toddlers under my table, and on babies while they were nursing. As long as I am physically comfortable, I can do the work.

A local master of the Irish accordion, a true son of Erin and deeply Catholic, was curious and a bit suspicious about CST. He asked, "Do I have to believe?" No. Animals and babies don't believe either, yet CST is effective for them.

Watching a CST session is about as exciting as watching grass grow. Search on www.youtube to see for yourself. If anyone you watch is making fast or forceful movements, they are not practicing CST. Remember the hallmark of CST is its gentleness.

The light touch characteristic of CST, five grams or less of weight, is the weight of a U.S. five-cent coin. My eyes close so that my hands open. I imagine energy flowing, like a scintillating band of light through my hands into the client. When I feel tissue motion, I focus my attention on it to get a sense of its pattern of movement and to evaluate its qualities. The tissue movements are subtle; they can be perceived by touch alone. One's skin is the sensing organ.

I once had a relationship with a wonderful bunny, a dwarf Hotot, Lara. We were friends. Like all rabbits, she was easily frightened. It took her months to feel safe with me; and she had to be reminded of that safety every day. I would hold her in my lap, touching only the tips of her fur, and imagine soothing her panicked breathing with the energy I sent from my hands through her fur into her core. After a while, I could feel her relax.

Today, years after her untimely death, I remember the feeling of soothing Lara with my hands while I am working, and I wait for a sense of inner turbulence calming. A deep breath, a sigh, a burst of heat or pulsation, or a cessation of the craniosacral rhythm are manifestations of this calming and are signs of tension release.

Once a pattern of tissue movement is felt, I can choose to either follow or resist it. My choice is based on my intuition, training, and assessment, my perspective. In my perspective, from my point of view, I am 100% correct. My perspective is unique and different from yours. We are both 100% correct from our own point of view. Two practitioners working on the same person have different perceptions; both are accurate and effective. This is one reason that the inter-rater reliability testing of CST is measured to be poor, although clients report relief. Two practitioners, both with hands on a client, will use CST differently, just as two physicians will treat an identical clinical situation slightly differently from each other, although their education and evaluations may be identical.

If all medical practitioners were identical, there would be no special doctors, none better or worse; it wouldn't matter who we saw. Individual variation is part of life, just as no two snowflakes are identical, yet all are five-pointed stars made of constant proportions of hydrogen and oxygen. It is the end result of the practitioner that matters. Is the client helped? Was the therapy effective?

When doing CST, my intention is for the greatest good for the dyad to emerge. I visualize what the anatomy under my hands looks like. I ask for guidance from the universe and from the bodies of the people on the table.

CST in the Scientific Literature

It takes motivation to learn, and effort to welcome and trust spontaneous and creative right-brained direction in therapeutic work. This has been difficult for me, trained as a registered nurse in the allopathic, mechanistic view of health. Doubts and questions about the value of visualizing, concerns about trusting intuition, and judgments about 'voodoo' emerged during learning, and are manifestations of left-brain dominance and the allopathic culture I was trained to follow.

The left brain wants therapy to be organized, concrete, and scientific. The right brain wants to 'go with the flow.' The left brain directs the musician to play all the notes and rests and accents correctly in a piece of music; the right brain puts in the passion that makes the music evoke an emotional response in the listener. The left-brain learns to read music notation; the right brain learns tunes by ear. It is best for both sides of our brain to work together, as both sides are equally valuable.

Thoughts About Observation and Judgments

Meridians and chakras are structures that belong both in the physical world and the energetic one. Both can be treated with CST, and both are difficult to measure with present technology. This could be one reason that mainstream research about CST has negative conclusions. A meta-analysis of 33 studies (Green, Martin, Bassett, & Kazanjian, 1999) concluded "this systemic review found insufficient evidence to support craniosacral therapy." Green commented that the seven studies showing the effectiveness of CST were low-level evidence. As CST is a relatively new modality, low-level evidence is where the evaluation process must begin. Another conclusion made by the authors is that current research methods have not yet been applied to CST using a large enough sample to prove or disprove effectiveness.

In the 1930s, some experts proved that bumblebees could not fly because their wings were too small in proportion to their bodies to generate enough lift. Of course, we see that bumblebees fly. The proof that they couldn't was a reflection of the understanding and evaluation skills of the time. It wasn't until the 1940s that researchers discovered that the four bumblebee wings function in a very different way from airplane wings (Pennicott, 2001).

In 2001, Chinese researchers used lasers to make accurate observations of bumblebees in flight. Seventy years after scientific experts proved that a bumblebee could not fly, there is now clear understanding of how bumblebee's wings work (Wilkinson, 1998). The point of this analogy about bumblebees is to appreciate that, in the future, a researcher will use an as yet heretofore unimagined technology to measure enough variables to prove what has been experienced and witnessed many times on a therapy table, that CST works.

PubMed, an organ of the National Institutes of Medicine, lists 29 citations for research studies about CST. CST has been found to be a "potentially useful adjunct" in the treatment of asthma.

Henci Goer, a published analyst of birth research, in a post to a maternity newsgroup stated, "A critical flaw in concepts of evidence-based medicine, from which flow other problems, is the premise that applying a set of rules to carry out studies and systematic reviews will produce an objective, reproducible, result, i.e., scientific Truth that can then be generally applied. But as long as studies are conceived, designed, carried out, and the results interpreted by human beings, their beliefs and biases will inevitably have influence every step of the way" (Goer, 2007).

How can the tools of observation and recording, valuing and measuring account for direct experience? How does one create a truly open experiment to determine what will happen? Like a self-fulfilling prophecy, an experiment designed to prove or disprove a null hypothesis unfolds differently to one that is spontaneous and dynamic.

If CST works and causes no harm, who needs to discover the reason? If it makes people feel better, it belongs in our toolbox. After treatment, the client can feel more involvement and control in her life; she can now act decisively in situations, instead of reacting. She is running her life instead of her life running her. In cases where breastfeeding is not recovered after CST, mothers report feeling much better and content because they have relaxed, let go of anguish, and discovered a renewed commitment and joy in their babies.

The question then becomes, "What is the value of CST? Maybe she would have gotten better after a massage." Perhaps that is true. There is so much that is unknown. There are too many questions. Perhaps the value in CST lies in the organization and confidence it gives to the practitioner? Or in the mindset of the person that has researched and chosen it? Or in the total focus given by the practitioner to the client? Oh, for unlimited research dollars!

How can one doubt the effectiveness of a gentle treatment when change is visible, as with a three-month-old diagnosed with reflux and colic by a pediatrician? This baby, the product of an induced labor, had long spells of crying (particularly after nursing). Breastfeeding was uncomfortable for mother and baby. Evaluation determined that the infant's parietal bones were overlapping her frontal bone, and that there was a kink in her dural tube, a torsion that was both irritating the nervous enervation to the gut and restricting the movement of the baby's pharynx and tongue.

During the cranial base release, the mother and I watched her breastfeeding baby's skull bones spread! The next day and during our follow-up, the mother reported a significant reduction in the frequency and duration of the crying spells and improved breastfeeding.

One report claims to show harm as the result of CST. This occurred in Holland, where a three-month-old baby girl died after her neck and back were forcefully hyper-flexed by the craniosacral therapist. Her breathing stopped, she had to be resuscitated, and she died as the result of complications. While craniosacral therapy has been blamed for this tragedy, the truth is that CST techniques are *never* forceful, and this practitioner was not following any of the principles or techniques that are the practice of CST. The Dutch CranioSacral Association denies that the manipulation performed by the therapist has anything to do with CST; furthermore, the Dutch Association does not recognize the therapist. Forceful manipulation has no place in CST (Holla, Ijland, Verlaat, van der Vliet, & Edwards, 2009).

Learning CST

The Upledger Institute offers two certifications in craniosacral therapy. Certification in CST techniques requires the applicant to complete 75 full ten-step protocols (the fundamental evaluation form that is taught to all beginners), to complete a techniques-level essay examination, an objective examination, and a practical examination where a master therapist is present to observe and to have hands on the same client as the applicant to evaluate treatment. The second certification, a higher level Diplomate certification, requires completion of a Diplomate-level essay examination, an objective examination, a practical examination, submission of five case histories, completion of at least 20 hours of a preceptorship program, and presentation of a six-hour presentation to an organized group or publication of an article.

As with lactation consulting, care is best when it is individualized. An excellent lactation consultant text (Caldwell & Turner-Maffei, 2003), describes six cases of mothers with identical symptoms: a hot, red, sore, and swollen breast. The reasons for the mastitis and its resolution are different for each case, even as the symptoms and presentation of all six are similar. "Craniosacral Therapy recognizes that no two people are exactly alike; that each treatment protocol is dictated by the wisdom of a person's own body; and that no two sessions are alike" (Upledger, 2005). Best practice means treating each dyad as unique.

Upledger training includes extensive education in anatomy because the more knowledge of anatomy one has, the better therapist one becomes. While working, the practitioner often imagines how the anatomy looks in that area. This practice serves to focus intention to put healing energies in the right places. Several case histories will illustrate.

While working on an eight-month, second-time pregnant woman who came for treatment to avoid a repeat of the misery that was her first labor, a vision came to me of her uterus and of her baby curled inside with a huge opening through her pelvis. It was like seeing inside her body. In due time, she had a lovely delivery with her second baby, who was in a right-occiput-anterior, perfect position. This was light years easier than her first three-day labor to deliver a baby presenting left-occiput-posterior. Can the difference be ascribed to CST, to a second-time labor, or to all the other things this mother did in search of a better labor? This mother reported that CST was enjoyable and provided relief from some of the discomforts of late pregnancy. In any case, it didn't hurt her or her baby.

In another case, while working on a client's foot and ankle, a vision came to me, like a waking dream image, of inside her ankle, with all its exquisite detail of muscle, bone, tendon, and ligament. At the same time, there was a regional tissue release, a burst of movement and release of heat, with a simultaneous awareness of general relaxation and comfort reported by the client.

Penny Simkin, P.T., in her 1995 video (*Comfort Techniques for Childbirth*) describes a technique to relieve back pain. This technique lends itself to CST application. When kneeling in front of a seated pregnant woman, resting my palms on her knees, I open my mind and wonder what the inside of her pelvic brim looks like. Many times images come to me of the inside of her pelvis. I describe what I see and often get validation of my impressions. "Yes, there was an injury on that side." "Yes, one leg is shorter."

Then I push my hands forward lightly, a nickel's weight at most, aiming her femurs straight back towards her lumbar region. I hold the pose, and the mother sighs and says, "Oh, that feels so good." We both perceive a shift in her pelvic/lumbar alignment. Her lower back pain is relieved. An observer would have seen nothing.

My First Big Case: Phyllis and Her Son

My first CST client (the one that set the hook deeply within me) was a physical therapist, whose pregnancy was uneventful, and whose labor and delivery was anything but.

Phyllis's labor began abruptly. The contractions quickly became long and violent enough for the midwife to nix plans for home delivery and send Phyllis to the hospital. A cesarean section delivered a baby boy tangled in the umbilical cord and floating in a meconium bath instead of clear amniotic fluid. He was intubated and deeply suctioned. Phyllis didn't get to hold him for six hours. He refused to latch in the hospital, despite multiple attempts. Phyllis was given a silicon nipple shield to facilitate breastfeeding. He lost 17 ounces by hospital discharge.

At home, she was able to manage some breastfeeding using the nipple shield, but it was painful, as her baby latched poorly. She established an abundant milk supply using a rental electric pump and regular simultaneous pumping. Her pattern was to endure 15 minutes of painful breastfeeding, and then she would pump and give her son three to five ounces via bottle.

When they came to see me at two weeks postpartum, the boy was gaining weight appropriately. Breastfeeding with the silicon nipple shield was still painful, although the shield fit her comfortably. His jaw was tilted, his mouth asymmetrical, and both his parietal bones were overlapping his temporal bones.

After some craniosacral therapy to the baby, he cried hard for a few minutes (in CST, this release of feelings is called *somatoemotional release*), and then lapsed into a deep sleep. The mother commented that she had never seen him relax so deeply during sleep before. His arms and legs were limp and externally rotated away from his torso. He slept deeply for about 20 minutes, woke up, started rooting, and then latched on to her bare breast comfortably and easily, (for the first time ever) and fed like he'd been doing it all his life. That was a magical session for me, and for the mother and baby, and completely sold me on the value of CST in breastfeeding rehabilitation.

After such a dramatic resolution, I expected instant results after CST with every client; the same mistake I made when I started using remedial co-bathing. It took time and clinical experience to learn that such miraculous resolutions are rare, are beyond anyone's control, that good comes from each session, and that there is nothing predictable in breastfeeding rehabilitation. Each dyad is different, with a unique process of recovery.

CST does only good. At a minimum, the client becomes more relaxed inside; at best, there is healing or recovery. There are few modalities that are as safe. I can think of none in the allopathic world with the safety of craniosacral therapy when performed as taught.

Mothers Receive Benefit from CST

A mother who is in pain, who is anxious, who can't sleep, who doubts herself or doubts breastfeeding is a candidate for CST, particularly if lactation management is proving ineffective or incomplete.

A birth that doesn't go the way she dreamed or where she has lost any control (Simkin, 1991) has impact on a mother. The impact may be physical. She may be injured or need to be sewed back together, or she may be left with residual backache. The impact may be psychic or emotional. She may suffer a crisis of confidence, and lose belief in her own abilities. She may feel that her baby is a stranger, even though she "knows" it is hers and takes excellent care of it. She may grieve the loss of the birth she wanted. She may be so focused on her own feelings, particularly if she is in pain, that she doesn't have energy to spare for her baby. All these experiences and feelings have an impact, usually negative, on breastfeeding.

What would happen to a relationship if you met the mate of your dreams, and within ten minutes of that meeting, were in a serious car accident? What would happen to that new love? Would there be time for lengthy telephone conversations, letters, and Facebook posts if you were hospitalized? For some women, a technologically driven birth is akin to an automobile accident or other traumatic event, like a friend who compared her unwanted induction/cesarean section with having her house burglarized. For love to grow, one has to have emotional energy to spare to develop and participate in the relationship. CST aims to help the dyad to heal, so there is energy to become fully engaged in the breastfeeding relationship.

One benefit of CST to the mother is the release of accumulated pelvic tension after birth. Postpartum mothers that I've worked with have all enjoyed pelvic diaphragm releases and sacral and lumbar work.

An example of a struggling dyad is the case of Adrienne who came for a consultation when her baby was nearly six months old. Her story was of a traumatic pregnancy, where her providers were negative and discouraging, and of a disturbing hospital course, where her desire for exclusive breastfeeding was undermined by staff attitudes and practice. Once home, she struggled with her baby to breastfeed, had milk supply problems, ended up pumping and bottle-feeding her milk, and would try every few days to put her baby to breast. The repeated failure to breastfeed alternately challenged and devastated her. Our session together was three hours long; her mood at the end was 180° different from that at the beginning. She went from almost expressionless to smiling and laughing as she left.

Once home, Adrienne chose to discontinue efforts to breastfeed, feeling ready to let go of that long struggle. She chose to continue pumping, feed her baby her pumped milk, let her baby start solids, and focus on having a good time with her baby. Would some other modality have yielded the same result? Possibly. Cognitive behavior therapy or a chiropractic adjustment or a counseling session with a religious authority or social worker might have all led to a similar outcome. Any dedicated practitioner of any modality where she was given all the time she needed to tell her story, receive some type of therapeutic touch to relieve body tension, and validation for her experience might have reached the same result. The CST blend of physical bodywork and energetic treatment is as valuable as any other manual therapy and deserves a place in the lactation therapist's toolbox.

Tips for Using CST with Dyads

When the dyad is breastfeeding, view and treat the mother and baby as two parts of one unit, as the recommendations given will have an impact on the mother and her baby in their mutually interactive, synchronous relationship. Dr. Christina Smillie refers to this synchrony as "the Mother-Baby Dance" in her lovely DVD of the same name. Synchrony is defined as "an essential component of the interaction between a mother and her infant, and is characterized by adaptive and reciprocal behaviors that promote a mutually rewarding interaction" (Reyna & Pickler, 2009). Clinically, synchrony means that mother and baby make a whole system, a dyad, where what is done with one partner of the dyad has an impact on the other partner, consequently affecting their relationship.

One goal is to calm the mother, so speak softly and create a healing environment. The calmed mother will move from the vigilance of sympathetic nervous system control to the calm receptivity of the parasympathetic one; the hormone shift favors milk flow. CST is one way to calm a mother, who then may relax enough to make more contact and improve communication with her baby.

The dyad's first session begins with CST for the mother. When the mother has no experience of CST and is relying on what she's read or been told, she is not 100% confident or safe with it. My experience has been that the mother has to feel comfortable with CST for it to have the maximum effect.

Using CST with the mother at the first visit has become routine in my practice. I learned this after a case where only the baby received CST. The mother watched her baby release tension, become soft and relax; then they had several comfortable breastfeeds in my office. When the consultation was over, the mother became obviously anxious, put her son in his car seat, and went home. In that night's follow-up telephone call, she reported the same breastfeeding problems that had brought her to me in the first place. She never came back for a follow-up visit. From that dyad, I learned that it is essential to work on the mother, so that she can feel the gentleness of CST, and from her own experience, serve as a platform to support her baby.

In several cases, the mother's level of anxiety has made it impossible for her to accept any suggestions, or to sustain any change for long. These cases have not had successful resolution. In one such situation, the mother and baby left after receiving CST combined with lactation consultation, only to call several days later, complaining that nothing I did was like anything the other lactation consultants she had seen had done, that nothing had worked, and expressing her displeasure. This visit was remarkable in that the mother never sat down, even attempting to breastfeed while standing. She was in constant motion during the visit and could not be calmed. Her displeasure with my work was a logical extension of her inability to relax, and my inability to calm her. Perhaps I was the wrong person to work with her; perhaps her issues were beyond my scope. One expert said that this mother was a classic picture of postpartum depression. In any case, CST did not get a chance to make any change, as she had but one treatment.

Mothers have to be prepared for the possibility of the baby having an emotional release. This was learned after a clinical fiasco. A mother came for CST for breastfeeding recovery. During the session, her son assumed the posture of a baby restrained on a circumcision board. He made the same particular cry that I remembered from my work as a nurse in postpartum, assisting (more times than I wanted) at this surgery. From his posture and his cry, he appeared to be reliving the surgery. She packed up and left; she never returned telephone calls nor answered letters. As a result, each new client is prepared for the possibility of the baby releasing the emotions around their past experience before I start working.

Exceptional Cases

Disconnection: Susan and Richard

Susan and Richard are an example of the impact of technology on a breastfeeding relationship. Susan came for CST when her baby was nine weeks old, still wanting to breastfeed, and with only three weeks left of her maternity leave. Another lactation consultant, who had assisted Susan in building a full milk supply, had recommended CST.

Susan told the story of her hospital birth experience over the course of two and one-half hours on the table, weeping or sobbing for much of that time.

Susan did not want to be induced, yet deferred to the recommendation of her obstetrician. The induction was started 12 days before her due date. As her core intention of not wanting the induction opposed that of the obstetrician who ordered it, the induction failed. While the epidural was being placed for the cesarean section after the long, painful, and failed induction, she fainted. Susan was revived, felt like she and her baby were going to die, and the operation continued. The anesthesia was incomplete; she felt her baby being pulled out of her with such force that her body moved on the operating room table.

Her son had obvious physical abnormalities. As she was in a large teaching hospital, his unusual appearance quickly drew a mob of students and hospital staff to the operating room. She heard all of their comments, including the term "FLK" (an acronym for "funny looking kid"). He was whisked away to Intensive Care, despite being healthy and strong, with APGAR scores of nine and ten.

She didn't see him for hours. He was given two bottles of formula in the NICU before she got him. When it came time to breastfeed, she was given a silicon nipple shield that hurt because it was too small for her nipple. She pumped and bottle-fed. She tried breastfeeding with the shield; it was always painful.

Because of his congenital anomalies, she was discharged home to immediately embark on a series of consultant visits. She never got to stay home and rest to recover from major abdominal surgery and to establish breastfeeding. Richard never felt like her baby, even though she knew he was hers, and she did everything she was supposed to do for him, despite having difficulty reading his signs and signals.

They received three CST sessions until breastfeeding was recovered, and then they had one more visit for breastfeeding management. During the first treatment, we discovered that emotionally, she had not moved past the fainting episode in the operating room.

At the first follow-up telephone call, between the first and second visits, Susan described a new calmness in herself and that she had lost the feeling that "every day was a failure."

In addition to the CST, breastfeeding was rehabilitated by lots of skin-to-skin care, remedial co-bathing, and safe bed sharing. One goal was for her to surrender control over schedule to discover what her son wanted, to explore him, and give him an opportunity to reach out and find her in his own time.

Pain-free breastfeeding was established after three weeks of rehabilitation. Their new connection stayed strong under the stress of her returning to paid employment outside the home. Besides the improved breastfeeding, the best sign of recovery came about a month after our first visit, the day she proudly announced, "This is MY baby."

Hyperarousal: Mary

Some mothers, such as Mary, are so hyper-aroused after their hospital experience that they can't relax and enjoy their baby. Mary described her birth as "awful," while she told her story. She was given zero choice about anything during the entire labor and delivery. She was told: "We are inducing you on Tuesday." She accepted this, believing the obstetrician to be the expert. When the induction was started, she was told, "We are putting this tampon-like thing in your vagina to start your labor." After some hours she was told, "Since you are dilating too slowly, we're putting this balloon-like thing in your cervix that will come out when you have gotten to three centimeters." At three centimeters of dilatation, she was given intravenous Pitocin™.

The balloon-like thing weighed her cervix down, stretched it, and hurt. The one wonderful staff person with her went off-shift and was replaced by an "awful one." She lost count after at least 15 vaginal exams. After two hours of pushing (on her back, holding her own thighs to pull her legs back), she was told, "If you don't deliver after another hour of pushing, you're going to have a cesarean section." She did push her baby out; her hips were so broad that it was difficult for me to reach both iliac crests with my forearm during a decompression technique.

After he was born, he was put on her chest briefly, and then taken away. In the hospital, she followed all the rules about breastfeeding, including the use of a predetermined position, the use of a nursing pillow, holding her breast in a C-hold, and using rapid arm movement to make him latch. She believed she had to endure pain, so his attachment would be correct. Part of her distress was anger; how could her nipples be damaged when she was doing everything right?

At home, Mary continued to do what she had been taught. This meant setting an alarm every two hours at night, so she could wake him to breastfeed. She feared he would become dehydrated otherwise. Mary used the word "fighting" when describing breastfeeding and reported many feeds ending when both she and her baby were in tears.

The baby was winning the fight. Babies always do. If their reflexes, desires, and abilities are not honored, they either refuse to go to breast or injure their mothers. Many times, the mother quits the struggle and weans.

Mary asked, "How do I hold my baby?" I have encountered this question in the past year from several mothers. When I first heard it, I couldn't believe it. Women don't need to ask how to hold their books in school or a purse, but some feel unable to hold their baby without guidance. This is a new (and personally alarming) clinical finding.

Mary was unable to relax enough after a two and one-half-hour CST session to let her baby latch without controlling every move he made, in part because she was afraid of being hurt again and in part because she didn't believe that a baby could feed independently. Even after watching a DVD of babies self-attaching, she refused to believe that her baby had the same abilities. With some gentle guidance and encouragement with all the time in the world, the dyad had a feed during our session that was a noticeable improvement. She was unable to sustain the improvement at home.

Instead of returning for more CST, Mary volunteered to be the subject for a master class in breastfeeding lead by a local expert. She was able to breastfeed comfortably in class and again unable to replicate her experience at home. She believed that the problem was that she had not yet found the best lactation help. At our last contact, she was searching for yet another expert and refused another CST session.

When the possibility was raised that her birth was far more than just "awful," and she was told that the LC has seen the impact of the birth experience impair breastfeeding and be a source of distress to a mother, her response was to say, "Well, the birth wasn't great, and I've put that behind me. Now my problem is that I can't breastfeed by myself at home alone." Mary is correct in her perception and she has not met the person yet to reach her. Unfortunately, the person she needs to meet is herself, and I was either the wrong practitioner or CST was the wrong modality, although I wish that Mary would have stayed with it for longer than one visit.

Deeper Issues Emerging: The Case of KC

With another case, Katherine and her daughter, CST opened the door to deeper issues within.

Katherine delivered a baby weighing 5-pound 14-ounce by cesarean section because the baby was in a breech presentation. The baby weighed 5-pound, 7-ounce at hospital discharge, and 8-pound 2-ounce at five weeks of age, an acceptable 2-pound and 11-ounce gain. Katherine came for help because breastfeeding was very painful, with nipples that were deformed by the latch. The second lactation consultant she had seen suggested CST. Katherine had been pumping and feeding the baby using a variety of recommended methods: a cup, finger feeding, a syringe, a Haberman™ feeder, and an Avent™ bottle.

This dyad came to my office at nine weeks postpartum. Katherine and her baby each received CST. The mother and LC cooperatively developed a care plan for home breastfeeding management.

Their strengths were that the baby was happy to go to breast, the mother was dedicated, and she had ample milk production. The care plan was that the mother was to avoid stuffing her breast into the baby's mouth. Instead, she was to position the baby so the baby could gape wide, with the lower lip as far away from the base of the nipple as possible. The baby was to be given the opportunity to latch on herself once the mother was comfortably positioned. The mother was encouraged to take baths and sleep with the baby, with the goal of maximizing their mutual delight in each other. Katherine was also encouraged to massage her baby. As she complained of excessive tiredness, she was encouraged to spend a day or two in bed, resting, even if this meant pumping, with the dad feeding an occasional bottle of expressed breastmilk. The mother made another appointment for CST in a few weeks; meanwhile, the LC stayed in contact with the dyad by telephone.

During the next 18 days, Katherine was telephoned three times. Her oversupply was managed by the use of positions that used gravity to slow the milk flow and by doing two feeds on one breast before switching sides, aka 'block feeding.' The mother reported that breastfeeding was steadily improving, and that the pain during feeding was gone. However, Katherine was not happy with the improvement, an unusual and unexpected development.

At the second office visit three weeks later, the mother received more CST. Towards the end of the treatment, she volunteered that there was more going on with her than just breastfeeding difficulty. She had begun to have memories surfacing about sexual abuse by a close family member when she was a small child. These old feelings were a burden in her present life with her new baby. Her feelings were accepted and validated, she was given support and empathy, and she was referred to several counseling services. Now the reason for her continued discontent, despite breastfeeding recovery, was clear.

In this case, CST was instrumental in getting to the crux of the mothering difficulty and directing the mother towards the help she needed. The peace and deep relaxation that was the result of CST created an environment where the mother could both increase her self-awareness and express what she learned about herself to the practitioner.

Torticollis: Sally and Jessie

The baby that is a candidate for CST is one with problems feeding, who is fussy or colicky, or who has a birth injury. A baby with an asymmetrical face or head, some restriction in movement, or a torticollis may also benefit from CST (Wall & Glass, 2006).

Torticollis is a contraction, often spasmodic, of the muscles of the neck, particularly the sternocleidomastoid, chiefly those supplied by the spinal accessory nerve. The head is drawn to one side and usually rotated, so the chin points to the other side. This makes comfortable breastfeeding difficult. Sally brought her baby girl, Jessie, born on June 10, to my office on August 23.

Jessie had an official diagnosis of torticollis and had been treated by a physical therapist for nearly two months, with no resolution. Sally, a nurse, did everything she was told to do (daily sets of strengthening and stretching exercises, and positional changes to induce symmetry) for her baby, even when the exercises made her baby cry. Sally came for CST as a last resort because her baby was still crying during the physical therapy, breastfeeding was still difficult due to the baby's restricted mobility, and the first lactation consultant she had seen recommended CST.

Jessie was a second baby; her older sibling had been breastfed for 20 months. Sally complained of difficulty breastfeeding because Jessie couldn't turn her face to the right side and didn't use her tongue in a comfortable way. As a result of the torticollis, Jessie preferred her right side for sleeping and eating.

Sally and I spoke on the phone several times before she came to see me. When we first met in my office, we spent time chatting before she lay down on my table, skin-to-skin with her baby, whose head was turned, resting on her right cheek, head facing to the left. Any attempt to turn Jessie's head was met with crying and active resistance. I stood at Sally's feet, with my hands cupping her heels, and lifted them gently. The craniosacral rhythm was evaluated and a still point induced.

After a few minutes, Sally sighed and her rate of breathing slowed. She started to tell the story of Jessie's birth. She had felt like a bystander in her own labor, as none of her wishes were honored. She wanted to be upright; she was told to lie down. She was hungry; she was denied food. She was thirsty; she was told the IV was enough and given only ice chips. She wanted to move about and change her position in labor; she was confined to bed and told to stay in one position, so the fetal monitor tracing would be clear. She spoke at length about her feelings as a result of being ignored by the doctor and nurses attending her. The actual delivery was wrenching and painful, despite the epidural, as the baby was born with a face-up presentation. Sally's emotions released in a torrent of words and sobs.

As Sally finished her story, Jessie woke and began to whimper. The whimper escalated to 20 minutes of crying, during which Jessie lifted her head spontaneously, turned it to midline, and put her face down on her mother's sternum, forehead resting there, and continued to cry. The torticollis released in front of our eyes, and the baby fell into a deep and immobile sleep. The baby slept for about 20 minutes.

When the baby awoke, she started seeking behaviors. Jessie went through all the steps of delivery self-attachment, but birth, as documented by Dr. Anne-Marie Widstrom, namely: rest, familiarization, searching, finding, rooting, latching, suckling, and sleep (Widstrom et al., 2011). The torticollis was gone forever.

Mandibular asymmetry can be an early sign of torticollis and can lead to difficult latch, sore nipples, infant weight loss, and diminished milk supply (Wall & Glass, 2006). It is interesting that in their report of 11 cases, ten of the mothers had complications of labor and delivery. The common symptom in all 11 cases was the infant's lower jaw tilt and difficulty latching. Wall and Glass suggest referral to an occupational or physical therapist for treatment; they mention chiropractic treatment and craniosacral therapy, which are also reported as effective options by parents.

Cathartic Triad of Behaviors

During years of clinical practice, a recurrent pattern of three infant behaviors has been observed, called the *cathartic triad of behaviors*. The three behaviors occur in a predictable cycle; in order, the behaviors are **r**oot, somatoemotional **r**elease, and **r**est—the 3-Rs. Babies that are put skin-to-skin will sometimes display these cycles spontaneously; I have seen this happen in the postpartum ward. When the concept was first introduced on an international listserve (LACTNET), many nurses, midwives, and lactation professionals wrote to me to validate the pattern. Five or six cycles of 3-Rs are the most that have been observed to date; two or three is most common.

There is no way to predict when a baby will manifest the cathartic triad of root, release, and rest. When babies express emotion in the hospital, they are often quickly quieted; a pacifier is put in their mouths or they are cuddled, swaddled or rocked. While the instinct to comfort a crying baby is powerful, I believe that if the listener has lots of experience and knows infant language, it is safe to let the infant express itself. The baby tells its story, just as "talking it out" is part of integration for adults. Adults talk to friends and family about their toothache, car accident, divorce, or about trying to find the right shoes for their kid. Freud is one of many who are famous for writing about the value of talking in therapy as the road to healing. If we have an accident or upset, talking about it is a relief; then we feel better and move on. Babies are people, too, and feel better after telling their story to the one person who cares most for them, their mothers.

Coach Linda Smith, BS, FACCE, IBCLC, FILCA, has been quoted for her basic rules of working with dyads. Ms. Smith's third rule is "It's her baby" (Smith, 2010). Keep this in mind while working. If the mother becomes uncomfortable and unwilling to let her baby continue to express emotion, and she wants to comfort her baby, support her. It's her baby. Tell her this at the outset. Give her all the control. Let her learn. You are only there as a guide to give practical advice and encouragement.

The cathartic triad of behaviors can mystify or frighten healthcare workers. Having presented "Babies Tell Their Stories" at lactation conferences, some of the feedback that I "like babies to cry" has been personally painful. This is despite clarifying the difference between seemingly random crying and a story being told. All infant crying is purposeful; it's just that we can't always interpret what the baby is saying.

Mothers who come for breastfeeding help benefit by practical advice and encouragement to follow their hearts, despite generations of cultural beliefs that babies have no feelings. CST is helpful in this regard. Perhaps it is the calm acceptance of the emotional outburst on the part of the practitioner that serves as a model? Perhaps it is that CST creates an atmosphere of sanctuary, where the important questions can be asked?

Know what distinguishes the cathartic triad from other types of crying. When the baby is skin-to-skin, most frequently the baby goes into deep sleep or self-attachment behaviors emerge. The baby will move, seeking the breast, and get close enough to latch. *When a cathartic triad is triggered, the baby* could *latch, but* won't. The baby's lips could be one hair's distance from the nipple, but the baby will NOT grasp it. The baby will instead have a powerful outburst of emotion. The listener can sometimes hear rage. Babies can get red in the face and pound their fists on the mother's chest, and cry so hard for a sob or two that they can hardly breathe. At other times, the crying has a pathetic or wounded quality. Mothers have to be prepared in advance for the baby's release of emotion. Once the baby starts to tell its story, encourage the mother to engage with her baby by saying things like, "Oooh, I didn't know that happened to you" or "Tell me more." Once the dyad establishes a vocal relationship with each other, breastfeeding is on the way to recovery.

After rooting and release, the baby will rest, reminiscent of the rest periods identified by Dr. Widstrom (Widstrom et al., 2011) After the rest, the baby may seek the breast again, and start another cycle of cathartic behaviors, or seek the breast, attach, and start breastfeeding. Mothers need steady and gentle encouragement and guidance while their baby is telling its story. Most become fascinated and start coaxing and supporting their babies, saying things like, "And then what happened?" or "I'm sorry it was so hard for you." or "Oh, I remember that." Witnessing this experience is a privilege, moving and sacred.

Babies can experience multiple episodes of forced latch, still practiced in hospitals, where the back of the baby's head is shoved onto the breast with the mother's nipple stuffed into the baby's mouth. Once latched on, sometimes mothers will hold their baby's head firmly in place, despite any infant squirming. Babies can be awakened from deep sleep and made to breastfeed. Often, healthy babies are taken away from their mothers at birth, a common practice that is completely without supporting evidence. Babies have reactions to all these events, just as an adult does when our desires are thwarted or we are injured.

While it is impossible, short of audiospectrographic analysis, to know precisely what the cries mean, one can speculate when looking at the whole cycle in context, linking the infant sounds with infant behavior. It would be wonderful to research this further, to use audiospectrographic analysis to catalogue the range of infant sounds, and link it with clinical outcomes.

The author feels confident, based on years of clinical observation, in saying that breastfeeding will improve once a baby has told its story.

The first time I observed a cathartic triad of behaviors was with the mother of a ten-day-old baby where remedial co-bathing was the strategy used to create a safe and intimate environment for the mother and baby. Up until then, they had never breastfed, although the mother had induced a full milk supply. The baby was thriving and getting nothing but her mothers' milk via bottle. Once in the tub, and after a few minutes of relaxing and getting comfortable, the little girl crawled to the breast and rooted. The mother had started leaking milk. The mother and I got excited, hoping to see the miracle of self-attachment. We were both surprised when the baby girl stopped rooting, even though her face was on the nipple/areolar complex. She began wailing and crying. Red-faced, she cried hard for about ten minutes, while I knelt next to the bathtub, feeling worried and anxious, sweat pouring down the back of my neck, imagining the mother becoming furious with me, and having no idea what to do. We both sat quietly and watched.

Perhaps my personal experiences in Primal™ therapy gave me a foundation of trust and familiarity with the noise–the baby's cries were reminiscent of the cries adults give when releasing powerful emotions. Primal™ therapy's gift is the wonderful and life-improving flashes of illumination and wisdom that occur once the energy of the old feeling is released. I had learned that release of emotion brought healing and recognized a similar essence in the baby's cries. The end result of the infant's cathartic triad was immediate and full breastfeeding recovery, a learning gift given to me early in my clinical career.

The second time a client's baby in skin-to-skin started to cry, memory of the first experience enabled me to stay calm. I encouraged the mother to stay calm by telling her that I had observed this behavior before. This particular baby had several cycles of the pattern of starting to crawl to breast, rooting, and then crying hard. In this instance, the baby did self-attach after the emotional release, doing parts of the self-attachment sequence: relaxation, grasping her mother's nipple and trying to bring it to her mouth, drooling, and eventually latching on unassisted.

Over the years, I have witnessed this triad of cathartic behaviors more times than can be counted, enough to help a new client not only listen to her baby, but also encourage the baby to tell its story. The exciting part of this triad of cathartic behaviors is that it always precedes breastfeeding, as if the natural process can resume once the baby has told its story (Lee, 2005). Megen J. Kuhn, RN, BSN, a nurse who has worked in NICU for over six years, has seen these behaviors, even with very immature babies (M. Kuhn, personal communication, February 24, 2011).

A baby that is releasing emotions around its history cries differently than a baby that is overwhelmed. The story-telling cries of emotional release reach a steady state (albeit a powerful one) and don't continue to intensify; the infant's body movements stay relatively organized and end after a few minutes, with the baby falling asleep. The overwhelmed infant's cries accelerate in tempo and intensity, along with increasing physical disorganization.

At present, we can only imagine what the babies are saying during a cathartic triad. As most common delivery and postpartum practices in hospitals in my region have no basis in evidence, it is easy to speculate that babies don't like those practices. Babies could be releasing feelings about their births, and their handling after the birth. Babies are often taken away from their mothers and handled in a detached, brusque manner by hospital staff that is doing a job instead of tenderly touching a new person. They want to breastfeed and can't. Babies are stuck with lancets and needles, circumcised, suctioned, and exposed to bright lights and cold. Babies are left alone. Dr.

Nils Berman, the South African neonatologist, travels the world speaking about the baby's reaction to being alone–the baby moves into sympathetic mode, fighting or freezing, having its survival mechanisms triggered, while waiting for mother to return.

Babies expressing their feelings vocally are often ignored or a pacifier is put into their mouths to silence them. How often has someone said that "they're too young to remember" when something painful is done to a baby? Dr. Henry J. Bigelow reported to the American Medical Association in 1848 that anesthetics were unnecessary for infants because they lacked the "remembrance of suffering." It wasn't until the 1970s that most infants were given anesthesia during surgery (Pernick, 1987).

Infants make a particular sound when they are speaking about the breast. In one conference session I presented, only one lactation consultant in a group of 30 was able to imitate this unique sound. Babies that expect their head to be shoved into the breast often have conflict about the breast. They really want it and they really don't, both at the same time. They've been conditioned to fear an unpleasant experience, yet their instincts draw them to the breast. Infants that both want and fear the breast will alternate between crying and making this special sound that I call, for want of a better term, the breast word.

Sometimes it is the baby and sometimes it is the mother who has the emotional release, as with Susan who cried for two and a half hours. Or Adrienne who clutched her naked baby to her naked chest and heart for three hours, as she told her story interspersed with spells of crying. After the emotional release, there has always been a change in the mother and in the baby. Resolution may mean a joyful weaning, as when Adrienne decided to stop the incessant pumping and bottle-feeding rat race and instead focus on skin-and-skin and fun. Or it may mean a delightful breastfeeding recovery. In either case, the dyad will do what is best for them, while the tension and struggle that have heretofore been part of their relationship is diminished.

Some mothers have weaned after emotional release. Perhaps the baby's emotional expression scared the mother? Maybe she doesn't have the understanding or security within herself to accept that her baby has emotions? Or maybe she didn't really want to breastfeed? Or maybe she felt responsible for some of her baby's anguish? Or maybe she was ignored as a baby and can't bear to hear HER baby cry like that, as the cries stir up too much old pain? One can only speculate.

Swedish midwives have reported (K. Svensson, personal communication, 2010) of the benefits of putting the baby skin-to-skin on the mother's chest and letting the mother tell her story as another way to recover breastfeeding. The midwives sit and listen. Sitting and listening, and connecting mother and baby is simple, effective, and reliable.

Thankfully, I've never yet seen a mother and baby having an emotional release simultaneously. That's probably a protective mechanism. If it happens, I must trust the process, stay calm, and keep my hands on lightly. I am ready.

Witnessing a baby releasing emotion can be anxiety-producing, unless one has sufficient experience. A client told the story of her three-week-old baby, hospitalized in a local teaching hospital's NICU to receive intravenous antibiotic therapy. The mother stayed with her baby, day and night, to hold and to breastfeed. One night, two nurses actively discouraged the mother from holding her baby. "Your baby needs to learn to cry," the mother was told. Vulnerable to the "expert" advice, she followed the recommendation. The baby cried all that night, except when she was being breastfed. The next day, a pediatrician recommended that the baby have a spinal tap because of concerns about her "irritability." Fortunately, the mother had the intelligence and strength to refuse.

As with a doula or midwife, who accepts and encourages the laboring woman's expressions of hard work and distress during labor, the CST practitioner accepts and encourages the story to be told. The release of emotions around an event enables healing; this is true in psychological counseling and it is true in craniosacral therapy.

There are times when CST hasn't worked, even when breastfeeding has been initiated comfortably, after the baby has had the emotional release and gone to breast, or when the clinical symptoms that brought the client for therapy have been resolved. These are the mysteries of clinical practice.

The first time a mother bailed out after beautiful breastfeeding was a shock to me. The dyad was left in their bedroom, tucked safely into bed together, having recovered easy breastfeeding. In the follow-up call the next day, the mother said that she weaned, that breastfeeding was not for her.

Release takes many forms and is different for each dyad. The dramatic releases, such as the mother that sobbed for most of the two and one-half hours of her first visit, have happened enough that this author has come to expect them. (A mistake-when will I ever learn?) Other mothers are more private with emotional release in front of a stranger. Some mothers will have a release that is subtle or even deferred until she gets home alone and has privacy to process her feelings. She will still benefit from CST.

Choosing CST Over Another Modality

I have thought long and hard about how to give guidelines. As this is a new area for lactation professionals, guidelines will become clearer over time, as more people discover and develop a clinical body of evidence. Sometimes the breastfeeding challenge is a symptom of something bigger than a breastfeeding problem.

If the baby is lacking an essential reflex, it should see an infant feeding specialist or medical specialist first before receiving CST. It is not within my scope of practice to diagnose any medical condition. The lactation provider can learn a lot by going with the mother to see the specialist. This is an educational excursion and will help different practitioners, in this case the infant feeding specialist and the craniosacral therapist or lactation consultant, create networks.

A recent client told me that an IBCLC she had seen told her that her baby had an aversion to swallowing, and would eventually learn to swallow. Swallowing is an involuntary reflex for a newborn, who cannot eat without swallowing. It is not something that a baby chooses to do or not do. The mother called for CST. After she described the infant's feeding patterns, she was referred to an infant feeding center. Lactation specialists need to be aware of their clinical limitations, and alert to the fact that a problem with feeding may not always be a breastfeeding problem.

At nine weeks postpartum, this mother had seen a number of lactation workers. Her baby took nearly an hour to feed at every feeding. She was pumping and giving her milk in other ways. Her baby was being fed with a tube-feeding device at breast or taped to a finger. He did things with his tongue that hurt her nipples. He was unable to take a bottle in the hospital. Time spent with this baby was detracting from her other children and her family life. She was exhausted.

She was given several referrals to infant feeding specialists. She was relieved because after nursing other children for years, she *knew* there was something not right with this baby, she could *feel* it. Clipping his tongue-tie didn't improve things enough, although she was meticulous about the follow-up tongue exercises. She was told that CST would still be appropriate as an adjunct therapy once she had a diagnosis, so she called me for an appointment. She was referred to an infant feeding specialist because my scope of practice does not include diagnosis. Once this baby received a diagnosis of torticollis, I was happy to provide CST.

Some lactation therapists have described clinical success stories where CST was helpful for babies after frenulotomy or who had high arched palates.

It is the practitioner's responsibility to practice wisely and with all intention for the highest level of safety and healing. This means sustaining follow-up until there has been either a resolution or another skilled practitioner takes on the clinical responsibility for management.

Barriers in Practice

As with lactation work, there is a resistance to having more than one visit with the practitioner. This makes no sense.

Imagine having a medical condition. Is it realistic to expect resolution after one visit with the provider? On the contrary, several visits need to be made to determine if the medication and its dose are working, make changes, and offer new recommendations. How then is it practical to have one lactation visit or one craniosacral therapy visit? Yet many people do that, and expect some magic to occur, if not immediately, at least within 24 hours. They may spend time struggling, while refusing to come back, or they may give up after insufficient treatment and tell their friends the modality didn't work. This is personally upsetting. In my experience, three or four visits are usually sufficient.

Another barrier is a fundamental disbelief in the modality. Modern culture in the U.S. generally does not value touch or energy medicine. Most hospital personnel touch mothers and babies with gloved hands. Nurses no longer give backrubs as part of routine evening care. Lab tests and monitors are the instruments of assessment, not the human hand. In the 21st century, many Intensive Care Nurseries do not practice routine skin-to-skin care. Some providers dismiss CAM. The good news is that change is coming.

Insurance company policies can be a barrier. Many people will not engage in any treatment if insurance will not pay for it; this is also true for lactation work. How many times do lactation consultants beat their heads against the wall, lamenting that a client will wean and go on to spend more money on formula purchases over the next year than would have been spent on a consultation or two? The consultation very well could have saved breastfeeding and given substantial return on investment. Some insurance companies will reimburse for only one lactation visit, when several are indicated.

Disagreement among healthcare workers is another barrier. Providers that have the most authority can either recommend or discourage consultation with the provider of a different modality. An example in current lactation practice is seen in the treatment of ankyloglossia. In my region, providers in one major health system forbid lactation consultants in that system to ever use the term "tongue-tie" with a client. Never mind what the evidence says, or what is clearly visible to the mother, or how her nipples feel. This type of discouragement is a barrier when clients ask about referral to any of the practitioners of CAM or to lactation consultants.

Finding a CST Practitioner

To find a reputable practitioner, ask in your neighborhood. Word of mouth is always an excellent recommendation. Another way is to click on 'find a therapist' on the home page of www.upledger.com and search by zip code. Everyone that has taken any Upledger training is listed on this page. Many licensed healthcare professionals attend trainings–medical doctors, osteopaths, dentists, physical therapists, nurses, occupational therapists and massage therapists. Find one in your area that has taken at least several Upledger courses. A curious person takes one course and never comes back; those that are truly interested and likely to be most helpful are those who have taken several courses and/or been a teaching assistant.

Clinical Tips

Potential clients are suggested to take three CST sessions. If it hasn't made any improvement by three visits, then either the modality is wrong or the practitioner is wrong for that situation.

Keeping calm, staying grounded, and feeling confident can be a challenge for the practitioner, especially at the beginning of integrating emotional release techniques into lactation practice. Sometimes one can feel shaky when realizing that the mother is paying you to help, and her baby is freaking out. If one chooses to use this technique, one needs an awareness and trust in the process that comes from personal experience.

As far as I know, there are no reported cases of using CST in an adoptive situation or cases of insufficient milk supply. These are clinical frontiers.

Sometimes recovery can be wonderfully dramatic, right in front of my eyes. Other times, the dyad leaves, the mother is amazed that three hours have passed, and breastfeeding still isn't reliable. Give it a few days. Sometimes the improvement is steady and slow, and the practitioner is the one to point it out to the mother. Other times, nothing gets better for a week or two, then BOOM! They are breastfeeding. Or if they aren't, they are much happier with themselves and getting along with each other better.

Sometimes the dyad will need to be left alone for a few days. Many times, breastfeeding gets so good that it seems the mother forgets she ever had a problem or perhaps she doesn't want to remember the hard times. When I have called, after a week or ten days, things are often improved, and the mother is cheerful. Relax if the mother doesn't answer the telephone or respond to an email after a few days or a week. Give them some time and space.

Dee Kassing. B.S., MLS, IBCLC, a lactation consultant in private practice, tells her clients to "expect to see some change in postural issues, such as if the baby looks like a crescent moon when lying on her back, she will probably be able to lie straighter after the first CST visit, or if she couldn't turn her head very far to one side, she will do better at it. Sucking is rarely affected by the first visit of CST… there will either be NO change at all in sucking after first visit, or there will be *one* wonderfully better nursing session, but then everything will be back to the way it has been. After the second visit, the mother should start to see some changes to suck, though it often still won't be perfect, or it might be perfect for a day or two, but won't hold, and the baby will have to go back again."

The reader is reminded that these anecdotes are the lowest level of research. However, there are enough of them that attest to the value of adding CST to our lactation therapy toolbox.

Remedial Co-Bathing

My first venture into remedial co-bathing, or putting mother and baby in a bathtub together, came after reading the work of Australian midwife and relief worker, Heather Harris (Harris, 1994). Her article and videotape released the same year, *Mandy and Matt: A Solution for Breastfeeding Attachment Through Co-Bathing*[31] were presented at an ILCA conference. Her work is cited by reputable researchers (Barbara Morrison RN, PhD and Gene Cranston Anderson RN, PhD, to name but two), but alas, it hasn't been replicated in any study, thus remaining officially unproven to the scientific world.

Ms. Harris drew upon nursing and imprinting research for the inspiration to combine skin-to-skin care with immersion in a tub of warm water. Her goal was to recreate, as much as possible, the initial meeting that should have occurred after delivery in order to give the mother and infant a chance to start over with each other. She described a typical immediate perinatal period as one of "noise, interference, and separation" that leads to "attachment difficulties and feeding problems" (Harris, 1994). Remedial co-bathing is a way for the "mother and baby to re-trace their steps and reclaim the quiet intimacy together they may have been denied at their birth" (Harris, 1994). Remedial co-bathing aims to restore connection on the dyad's timetable, with the attendant keeping a low profile. Ms. Harris makes the wonderful comment, "Even if the bathing does not end in a breastfeed, it is not a failure, as invariably both mother and baby will have received immense emotional nourishment from each other" (Harris, 1994).

Learning from Experience

The first time I used remedial co-bathing clinically was in 1995. The baby had not breastfeed at all prior to discharge from the maternity unit. The mother had started using a hospital-grade electric pump regularly in the hospital; her baby was thriving being bottle-fed her mother's milk. Our appointment together was on postpartum day ten.

The mother was open to remedial co-bathing once it was presented as something new to try. We went to the bathroom and filled the tub with comfortably warm water. The only light was from candles. The baby was placed on her mother's abdomen, partly immersed.

---

31   https://www.birthinternational.com/products/digital-video-disc/mandy-and-matt-dvd

After a few minutes, the baby began to crawl towards a breast, stopped, cried for a minute, and then rested. She repeated that sequence a few times, gradually reaching an areola. The mother's milk supply was so ample that she started leaking as soon as the baby was put skin to skin. Once the baby reached the areola, she lay there, taking an occasional lick of leaked milk. The mother used a cup to drizzle bath water over her baby for warmth. After half an hour, the baby's skin turned mottled which meant she was getting cold. The mother handed the baby to me, got out of the tub, dried herself, and then dried her baby.

What happened next was a miracle. I was still floating an inch off the ground a day later.

After they were dried, the baby, still wrapped in a towel, started showing feeding cues. The mother opened her bathrobe, put the baby to breast, and that little girl latched on as if she been breastfeeding all her life. At one month postpartum, they were breastfeeding easily and happily. All after one session in the tub!

This dyad's dramatic breastfeeding recovery was the first immediate resolution of a breastfeeding problem I had ever witnessed. It demonstrated that remedial co-bathing could be a useful technique in breastfeeding rehabilitation and showed me the value of skin-to-skin as a therapeutic tool. (It was also the first glimpse of the cathartic triad of behaviors described in the chapter on craniosacral therapy.)

As remedial co-bathing had worked so well, I began to use it in every consultation, seeing it as a magic tool to fix any breastfeeding problem. That was a mistake. It is a mistake to rely on only one strategy as "the answer" for every situation. Another mistake is to create an expectation that the bath will absolutely fix breastfeeding. If the co-bathing doesn't work, the mother is disappointed and the breastfeeding therapist loses credibility. It is best to present co-bathing as something new and fun to do with the baby.

Not every mother will relax and feel comfortable being naked in a bath with her baby, while the lactation therapist, a stranger, is watching. As the mother's comfort is important, the practitioner must be sure the mother gives full consent. If the mother shows any hesitation or reluctance, then use another strategy.

In one case, I coaxed the mother into remedial co-bathing, presenting it as *the* way to recover breastfeeding. The mother and baby spent a long time in the tub, and there was no resolution of the breastfeeding difficulty. In retrospect, this particular mother was neither completely open to nor comfortable with this plan, but deferred to the authority of the hired lactation "expert." Her questions and doubtfulness were over-ridden by the overly enthusiastic practitioner (me). Her reticence should have been honored and another strategy found, or she could have been given time to think about it, instead of being pressured into doing it right then and there. The LC has to build and sustain trust and credibility; presenting a strategy outside the mother's experience or comfort zone requires time for consideration and discussion.

One client, a 42-year old partner in a law firm, was stunned into joyful, awed silence when her baby latched on in the bath. "She wants me," were the first words out of this mother's mouth, accompanied by tears of wonder and delight. She enjoyed co-bathing so much that for the first week after our visit, she took three baths a day! She loved seeing her baby reach out to her, and greatly enjoyed the self-attachment, and the sensual aspect of her baby's warm soft skin. After six years of fertility interventions, a miserable pregnancy, an induction, a cesarean section, and the surprise of actually having a real live baby after years of struggle, expense, and stress, the mothering role was a surprising challenge. For her, the bath was about fun and learning the intimacy that is part of the breastfeeding relationship. This was completely foreign to her achievements as a partner in a law firm. For her, the easy simplicity of being in a tub of warm water with her baby was priceless.

When to Use Remedial Co-Bathing

When a mother wants to breastfeed and can't, she is not happy and not having much fun with her baby. The unhappiness can be amplified by an intensive lactation recovery prescription that may include a sequence of pumping both breasts for ten or 15 minutes, trying the baby at breast (sometimes with a nipple shield and/or a tube-feeding device or periodontal syringe), and bottle- or finger-feeding the pumped milk. This whole sequence might be repeated at least eight times in 24 hours. When a mother is working all the time to sustain milk supply and to feed her baby, when does she have time for the rest of her life: sleeping, eating, showering, taking care of her house and family (which can include other children), and enjoying the baby? Vigorous lactation routines can lead to premature weaning because there is little fun or pleasure to balance the hard work. In some cases, there is an additional pressure of time, as the mother may feel an urgency to establish breastfeeding before the specific date to return to employment outside the home.

Remedial co-bathing is a way to offset that work and pressure with something easy and relaxing. The mother can have some sweet time, cuddling and counting toes without focusing on her breasts and milk production. Remedial co-bathing can lighten the atmosphere, reduce tension, and reinforce that fun is an essential part of mothering.

Remedial co-bathing can signal the beginning of an important shift in the dyad's relationship, where the mother lets go of the administrator role. Instead of counting, measuring, pumping, and feeding, she begins to embrace her baby, and starts stroking, sniffing, and grooming. She lets go of 'nurse' and becomes 'mother.'

Remedial co-bathing can be a way for a dyad to connect when a mother is resistant to being skin-to-skin. In such cases, skin-to-skin will make sense to her because no one wears clothes in the bath.

"High-touch and low-tech" is the way Ms. Harris has aptly described remedial co-bathing. In today's era, where anything new usually means a purchase, it is wonderful to offer mothers a strategy that can be done immediately with resources already available in their home.

Important Tips

It works best to present remedial co-bathing as something fun for a mother and baby to do together, with no mention of its potential to help breastfeeding. Encourage the mother by saying something like, "Let's see what happens." or "I wonder what your baby will do." For a breastfeeding strategy to succeed, the mother must understand what is involved, what the pros and cons are, and she must be willing to participate with all her heart. If she has to fight her own belief system, there is a greater chance the strategy will not work. Her intention will be different from yours, making for a difficult consultation. Present the new idea, then give the mother a chance to think it over, discuss it with family and friends, and explore it on the Internet before the actual consultation.

Setting the Stage for Remedial Co-Bathing

Keep the lights low to replicate a womb environment. As some bathrooms have bright overhead lights, use candles to provide dim light. Or have lights on in a room next to the bathroom and leave the bathroom door ajar.

Maintain privacy. Arrangements may need to be made for the care of other children.

The bathroom should be warm. The water temperature should be warm, between 98 and 102 degrees F, comfortable to both mother and baby. Running a trickle of hot water into the tub keeps the water warm for the entire bath time. Remember to let some water out periodically to avoid a flood.

Bring a cup or small bowl to drizzle bath water over the baby to keep it warm.

The mother may enjoy having a cool wet washcloth to wipe her face, as snuggling in warm water with a warm baby can make her feel hot.

Keep a drink of the mother's choice within easy reach.

Prepare the mother for her baby to tell a story. Some babies will start crawling to the breast, then stop and cry, then rest. (This is the cathartic triad of behaviors discussed in the craniosacral therapy chapter.) Encourage her to listen to and talk with her baby. Sometimes a skilled practitioner may imagine out loud what the baby might be saying. Asking the mother to talk about the birth and their first days together may be helpful.

Suggest the mother use her arms as a friendly fence to keep the baby from falling off her torso.

Bring an armless chair next to the tub. The lactation therapist can sit on it (and save her knees!) and be comfortable. The mom can use the back of this chair as something to lean on when she is moving in and out of the tub. If the attendant sits on the chair, and the legs of the chair are up against the tub, the chair will not move and will give the mother strong and safe support.

Create a relaxed atmosphere, where there is time for the process to emerge on its own timetable.

Speak in soft tones. Use short sentences. Encourage the mother to focus on her baby.

For safety's sake, suggest that someone else be within easy call or reach of the mother in the tub if the mother wants to use this technique again. Use a bath mat in the tub to give her secure footing. Some mothers prefer to hand the wet baby over to another person during the transfer out of the tub.

Helping the Mother and Baby During and After the Bath

Sometimes babies will move to the breast to lick and nuzzle and explore at a leisurely pace. The challenge for the LC is to keep the mother from forcing the baby to the breast. Using her arm to R.A.M. (an acronym for Rapid Arm Movement) the baby onto her breast, or pushing her breast into the baby's mouth may be irresistible. She may have been taught to do this in the hospital, and it may have become deeply ingrained as part of the pattern she's been repeating, even though it has not helped breastfeeding, and, in fact, may have undermined it. Sometimes mothers have to be guided to make conscious decisions NOT to do what they have always done, which is to "latch the baby on" themselves. The LC may be tempted to "help" the baby, who may be so close to latching that it appears just the tiniest bit of assistance will make the latch happen. Sit on your hands!

It can be challenging and stressful for the LC to sit on her hands, watch, and wait, and let the baby take its own time, while the baby is mouthing the nipple and is only a hair away from grasping the breast. Healthcare professionals are not trained or encouraged to sit and observe; they are taught to do things, to intervene. This does not always work with babies or with breastfeeding. The goal in remedial co-bathing is for the dyad to discover their way of breastfeeding. When the LC sits on her hands, the best behavior is modeled for the mother, and the baby has the necessary opportunity to use its own abilities.

For many women, being naked in a tub of comfortably warm water is the height of luxury and relaxation. When a mother relaxes, her baby relaxes, too. They may both take a short snooze at this time. The average length of these restorative naps is about 15 minutes. The helper simply lounges next to the side of the tub and uses a cup to trickle warm water from the tub over the baby. Keep lights low; daylight is sufficient. Bright, flickering, overhead lights make babies retreat into a shell to avoid the intrusive glare. A candle is sufficient if no dim electric light is available. The room has to be warm. All are comfortable: mother, baby, and helper.

The lactation therapist's job is to be patient, coax, and reassure the mother as she enters the process of discovery of her baby's abilities and ways of communicating. Give her practical advice and encouragement to give control of the feed to the baby. New mothers may have very specific ideas for breastfeeding that they learned in childbirth class and read in books or on the Internet. The notion that her baby is as well equipped as a newborn kitten or puppy to self-attach is impossible for some women to believe until they see it themselves. Some women have laughed (always good for releasing tension) at hearing that all she has to do is set the table; it is her baby's job to pick up the fork.

"Let us remember that the bottom line is for the mother and baby to enjoy this event" (Harris, 1994).

Homeopathy

Homeopathy is a healing modality that is over 200 years old. The hallmark of homeopathy is its gentle and specific treatment for all the symptoms an individual presents—emotional and mental, as well as physical. Homeopathy is a leading therapy in Europe and Asia, particularly in India and countries that were part of the British Commonwealth.

History

Samuel Hahnemann, a German-born physician, is credited with the founding of homeopathy. He started experimenting with new methods and ideas of treatment in 1790 because he was turned off by the medical practice of the times, which included bloodletting, purging, and using harsh chemicals. At one point, he became so disillusioned with the medicine of the day that he gave up practicing medicine entirely and made his living by doing medical translations, as he was fluent in eight languages, including Latin and Greek. Dr. Hahnemann was the first to test drugs on healthy people to determine their effects and is considered to be the "father of experimental pharmacology" (Morrel, 2011).

Dr. Hahnemann's discoveries about the therapeutic use of substances appealed because of their gentleness and specificity. Homeopathy spread through Europe and was brought to the U.S. in the 1820s. Students founded the first homeopathic medical school in the late 1800s, which proved helpful in treating scarlet fever, typhoid fever, cholera, and yellow fever. In the early 1900s, homeopathic practices spread; there were 22 homeopathic medical schools and 100 homeopathic hospitals in the U.S. Boston University, Stanford University, and New York Medical College taught homeopathy.[32]

Several forces contributed to the decline in the popularity of homeopathy. One was a new organization, the American Medical Association (AMA), whose mission was to eliminate all other healing modalities, deeming them to be without merit because they lacked scientific foundation. The other was that new drugs were easier to give to more people. Homeopathic diagnosis takes a long time. Prescribing the same drug to everyone with a sore throat was easier and faster than identifying all the individual symptoms in each

---

32   www.wholehealthnow.com/homeopathy_info/history.html

person with a sore throat in order to find the precise remedy specific to that person.

As with other modalities suppressed by the AMA after the Flexner Report was released in 1910 (Flexner, 1910), another reason that homeopathy fell out of flavor was that physician training was changed to conform to a Germanic model, as Dr. Flexner was of German background and education. Today, skepticism about homeopathy (and midwifery, chiropractic, optometry, and podiatry) still lingers as result of this century-old campaign.

Homeopathy Today

Today, attitudes are changing. Some medical doctors are now calling individualization of treatment by the name 'differential therapeutics' and finding value in the approach (Merrell & Shalts, 2002). In a study examining the treatment of 30 children with upper respiratory infections, there were statistically significant differences in favor of homeopathy. Individualization of treatment was highlighted as a valuable and useful characteristic (Ramachandani, 2010).

Ninety-four percent of French pharmacists recommend homeopathic medicines to pregnant women (Damase-Michel, Vie, Lacroix, Lapeyre-Mestre, & Montastruc, 2004). The British Royal Family have used homeopathy for three generations,[33] and there are currently five homeopathic hospitals within the National Health Service, some with two-year waiting lists. About ten percent of German physicians specialize in the practice of homeopathy. Medical doctors in Switzerland, Italy, Russia, Spain, and the Netherlands either use homeopathy or refer to homeopathic practitioners. There is great acceptance and utilization of homeopathy by professionals and the public in these countries. "The Swiss Federal Office for Public Health issued a report to the government of Switzerland which concluded that 'the effectiveness of homeopathy can be supported by clinical evidence, and professional and adequate application be regarded as safe" (Bornhoft et al., 2006). Homeopathy is popular in South America and India, and has seen resurgence in popularity in the U.S., starting in the 1970s.

How Homeopathy Works

One theory is that the ultra-low doses of a substance stimulate the patient's body to react to the disease or condition, like vaccines (low doses of

---
33 http://www.my-homeopath.com/facts.html

the causative organism) stimulate an immune response. Dr. Hahneman discovered that substances inducing symptoms in large doses would relieve them in very small doses. He coined the classic phrase, *similia similibus currenter*, "like cures like" to describe this concept. For example, a large dose of ipecac induces nausea, salivation, and vomiting in a well person. Giving a homeopathic dose of *ipecacuanha* can relieve the sufferer of symptoms of nausea, salivation, and vomiting. Too much coffee keeps one awake, whereas the active brain trying to fall asleep can be helped by a homeopathic dose of *coffea*. Homeopathy is opposite of allopathy, which is "a system of therapeutics in which diseases are treated by producing a condition incompatible with or antagonistic to the condition to be cured or alleviated" (Lockie, 1989).

A homoeopathic practitioner (a nurse, physician, any licensed healthcare professional, or skilled layperson) will take several hours to learn the complete history and collect the details of all major symptoms. The range of questions asked is broad; for example, questions about pain include: location, type (throbbing, burning, stabbing, etc.), timing (what hour of the day or night), duration, frequency, associations (with environmental temperature, diet, movement, or emotion), what has relieved it, what brings it on, as well as recurrent thoughts, dreams, cravings, and feelings. When all the details of the patient's physical condition, and emotional and mental states, are organized into patterns, the practitioner then looks for a remedy that would induce that pattern if given to a well person.

Several styles of homeopathy have developed over the past two centuries: classical (where single remedies are used), constitutional (one high-potency remedy is used and the patient is monitored for change over a long period of time), combination (where remedies contain several ingredients), and complex (where remedies may contain up to 25 ingredients). The essence of the remedies, infinitesimal quantities of the substance, is unchanged. How they are combined and used is different, depending on the style of the practitioner.

The homeopathic history taking can be healing in and of itself. It is restorative and refreshing to tell all the details of one's story to an interested listener over the course of one or two hours. This is very different from a visit with a medical doctor, where the chief complaint is presented, physical assessment is done, some lab tests ordered, and medication is prescribed, all in an average of 15 or 20 minutes.

Someone going to the medical doctor for a sore throat and fever would have their temperature, pulse, and other vital signs measured by office staff. Then the doctor would perform a more thorough physical examination, looking in ears and throat, palpating the throat and neck, listening to the heart and lungs, and swabbing the throat to determine the causative organism. The patient would be asked how long the throat had been hurting and about any exposure to illness. Then prescriptions would be written to treat the suspected organism and to make the sore throat and fever go away.

A homeopathic practitioner might discover that the person with the sore throat and fever is also sensitive to light, is having profuse perspiration, and has a dry mouth and a red face, all characteristics of *belladonna*. Another person with a sore throat and fever could present with a swollen throat, and pain that is stinging and relieved by cold drinks, all characteristics of *apis mellifica*. Even though the chief complaint (sore throat and fever) is the same in both people, each clinical picture is different. The homeopathic treatment is specific and tailored to the individual.

How Homeopathic Remedies Are Made

Remedies come from actual plant or animal material, or specific minerals, salts, or foods. The material is soaked in an alcohol/water solution for a month. After that time, the solution is saturated with the chemical properties of the material and is now called a *mother tincture*. One drop of the mother tincture is added to nine drops of an alcohol/water mixture and is shaken with impact, or succussed, many times. One drop of this dilution is added to nine parts of an alcohol/water mixture. Dilutions to the power of ten give the X potencies. The dilution/succession process is repeated until the desired potency or strength is reached. By the time a 6X potency is reached, there is not enough of the original material in the remedy to cause any toxic effect, and the drop of mother tincture has been diluted 610 times. The healing properties of homeopathy come from the number of dilutions; the more dilutions, the stronger the remedy. The succession process refines and concentrates the energetic properties of the original substance.

C potencies are made in a similar manner, except that one drop of material is added to 99 drops of the diluting solution. Materials that won't dissolve in diluting solution, such as gold or aluminum, can be blended with sugar and crushed into powder using a mortar and pestle until they are fine enough to be dissolved in solution.

Once the final potency is reached, it can be blended with lactose to make tablets, sucrose to make pellets, or a cream or gel base to make an ointment. Remedies are usually put under the tongue to be dissolved, although they can be dissolved in water or human milk and given by spoon.[34]

---

34 www.classichomeopathy.com/remedies/howmade.html

X potencies are considered weaker than C potencies, stay in the body for a short length of time, and are useful in first aid, sudden illness, and seasonal problems.

C potencies up to 200 C are medium-strength potencies and are useful for more chronic health concerns. Highest strength potencies are 200 C and above, up to 10 M. Higher potencies can stay working in the body for months, and are useful in treating constitutional or hereditary conditions, such as allergies.[35]

An advantage to homeopathy is that anyone can learn enough to treat themselves and their families for most common illnesses, saving expense and time. Homeopathic remedies are relatively cheap, easy to find, and without harmful side effects, another advantage in this day and age of spiraling healthcare costs.

Conflict Between Allopathy and Homeopathy

An example of this conflict is manifested in a meta-analysis of homeopathy that showed the situation did improve, but didn't count. "Even though such a meta-analysis yielded a significantly positive result, with a combined odds ratio of 2.45 favoring homeopathic remedies over placebo, the conclusions that can be drawn from such a meta-analysis are limited and several caveats have been identified" (Ernst & Pittler, 1998). Such a conclusion is an example of a prevailing negative attitude about homeopathy; even though homeopathic treatment was effective, Ernst and Pittler are still skeptical.

There is a report of a homeopathic remedy, Gali-col, considered to be the cause of apparent life-threatening events in a number of Israeli infants (Aviner et al., 2010). Laboratory analysis of samples discovered the presence of ethanol, propanol, pentanol, glycerol, and sugars. These ingredients were not identified on the label and are not part of standard homeopathic compounding. Another problem was that parents of affected infants were not following dosing instructions on the label. Yet the implication in the article is that the homeopathic ingredients were the source of risk, rather than the manufacturing or the lack of adherence to proper dosing. Manufacturing problems and incorrect dosing are challenges in the use of any medication or remedy, and both contribute to at least 2,000 deaths from allopathic medications a year (Starfield, 2000).

---

35   http://www.elixirs.com/faq.htm

In a randomized clinical trial of homeopathic remedies done in Nicaragua, a statistical difference was found in length of diarrhea episodes and in number of diarrhea stools per day of treated infants (Jacobs, Jimenez, Gloyd, Gale, & Crothers, 1994). Criticism of this trial in subsequent letters to the editor of *Pediatrics* included the comment that different homeopathic remedies were used. As homeopathic remedies are prescribed on an individual basis, depending on the individual's particular symptoms, constitution, and feelings, the criticism is hardly fair.

In studies of allopathic medication, all subjects in a RCT receive either the medication or a similar-looking substance. The prescribers are unaware which medication they are administering. In the Nicaraguan study, each child was diagnosed and given an individualized homeopathic treatment, one of five remedies. In some cases, the remedy was a placebo, whereby some children received dummy remedies, unbeknownst to parent and provider, to meet the conditions of a double blind, randomized controlled clinical trial. When the study was over, the children that received the homeopathic remedies had significant improvement in their condition, recovering nearly a day faster than the control groups.

For two years after the Nicaraguan study was published, letters were written from both sides, one defending the modality and the other attacking it. Fisher and colleagues (Fisher, Dantas, & Reilly, 1996) made these comments: "There are significant numbers of doctors practicing homeopathy in many countries where diarrhea is a great public health problem... Sampson and London's critique of Jacobs et al.'s double-blind placebo-controlled clinical trial... is harsh, peremptory, and contrary to the scientific evidence." Jacobs responded (Jacobs, 1996) with a defense of the original study. In the same issue, Edward Chapman, MD, DHt, President of the American Institute of Homeopathy (Chapman, 1996) had this to say about the discussion, "The American Institute of Homeopathy has represented homeopathy to a skeptical medical profession since 1844. The general openness of medical professionals today to the positive outcomes being documented from homeopathic practice gives hope that the two world views can find a common ground in which patients receive the safest, most efficacious, and cost-effective care."

A meta-analysis found homeopathy to be effective in treatment of childhood diarrhea, fibrositis, hay fever, influenza, pain, side-effects of radio- or chemotherapy, sprains. and upper respiratory infection; this paper also calls for more research (Mathie, 2003).

Homeopathy in Lactation Practice

How might a lactation professional use homeopathy in clinical practice? Unless one is certified or trained, or it is within the scope of one's practice to prescribe, it would be best to refer. In my region, there are two homeopaths who are also pediatricians, a lovely combination for optimal patient care.

There are many remedies for the situations lactation professionals will encounter. *Lac Defloratum, Galega Off., Calcarea Phosphorus, Urtica Urens,* and *Ricinus communis* are all possibilities to consider when milk supply needs increasing. *Phytolacca* is useful in the treatment of some women with mastitis. *Conium* is useful in particular cases of breast pain. Homeopathic remedies are safe to take when nursing and will not have any impact on the nursing baby.[36]

As discovering the right remedy can be a painstaking and tedious process, the Internet offers some solutions. A Google search for "finding the right homeopathic remedy" yields over 639,000 sites. Taking care of one's health is not easy; however, the person who cares the most about personal health is that person. Surrendering health decisions to another person is a serious act. Taking charge of one's own healthcare takes time, education, and a willingness to keep exploring.

Some say that a placebo effect, and not the homeopathic remedy, improves the patient's condition. If that is true, where is the harm? The person is still relieved. However, infants and animals lack belief systems (at least to our current knowledge), and so are free of the cognition that would respond to a placebo; they respond well to homeopathy. In my role as camp nurse at a music and dance camp in upstate New York since 1980, I have given *ledum palustre* to small children in misery from bug bites, and *chamomilla* to teething infants. To see the child be relieved within one minute, fall into a deep sleep, and wake up happy is impressive and rewarding. To have children come look for me for more *ledum* also confirms homeopathy's value.

Homeopathic remedies are worth considering if a mother has mastitis or breast pain, or her baby has colic or teething. One can encourage a mother to explore homeopathy for herself. The wrong remedy will simply not work, so there is little risk to mother or baby. It is appropriate and wonderful for a mother to take care of her own family when dealing with acute self-limiting conditions, such as colds and poison ivy. Chronic conditions require a depth of knowledge to determine the best remedy and are best referred to a certified or licensed practitioner skilled in homeopathy.

36 http://www.otherhealth.com/homeopathy-discussion/814-homeopathic-remedy-increasing-milk-supply.html

Clinical Tips and Summary

I would like to share some clinical tips, based on successful clinical work, that don't fit into any other chapter.

At the End of the Visit

A mother with breastfeeding problems needs memory aids, as she can be overwhelmed by her newborn, her physical and emotional changes, her life alteration, and by breastfeeding. An overwhelmed mother has limited memory skills. She needs help to remember what she will change in her daily routine after the consultation.

At the end of the visit, interview her. Ask her what she will remember to do when you are not there. Ask her what helped during your visit. Write down her exact words on the care plan. Her words will trigger her memory more than any words of yours.

Once she is finished, and you have written up the care plan, have her read it back to you out loud. Make sure she can read your handwriting and that she understands her own words. Sometimes a little sketch is useful. Call her attention to where this care plan will be put. Make a note of its location in your chart. This will help both of you remember the details. Carbon or pressure-sensitive papers are useful to make copies.

Use her cell phone to take a photograph of mom and baby *comfortably* nursing. This is proof that she and her baby can breastfeed. If she did it once, she can do it again. Take the picture while she is nursing and is relaxed and mellow. When the nursing mother is glowing and relaxed, and smiling a little, it is a sign of oxytocin release and milk flow. It is her choice to be skin-to-skin or lightly clothed.

Use Her Support Network

When present, the mother's group of family and friends can learn a lot about breastfeeding by attending some of the consultation. They may remember things the mother won't or can't.

Teach them to offer her a drink when they notice her lips are dry. Asking the mother "do you want apple juice or water?" diverts energy from the mother who has to make a decision. Instead, give the mother a glass of water with a straw in it, and say, "Drink."

Ask her family and friends to help with shopping, cleaning, laundry, and housework. The mother's closest social network wants to do things to be helpful. Left to their own devices, they can usurp the baby or make the mother more anxious. Giving them useful things to do diverts their energy into useful channels. If a bris or some religious ceremony is planned in the first week postpartum, encourage the mother to select an event planner. I've encountered too many cases where a mother can't or won't focus on breastfeeding because she is coordinating a social event. When her focus eventually turns to breastfeeding, restoring connection is more difficult and may not go the way she dreamed.

Engage the support network in problem solving. Even when they can't identify the problem, asking for their involvement opens the doors for them to learn. They feel included, another good thing. It helps to know what they think and believe. Educating them will help the mother when you are not there.

Be prepared for the women in her network to want to talk to you about their own infant feeding experiences; listen with an empathetic ear. Once they've told their own stories, they will be more helpful to the mother, your client.

Competing Authorities

Sometimes mothers will have seen other lactation professionals before you. Maintain professional and collegial communication in such situations. Whatever complaints a mother may have about another practitioner are best going in one ear and out the other. What a mother hears and what was actually said are two different things. Remember that other practitioners will be seeing the mothers who are dissatisfied with you!

My choice is not to call another practitioner to inquire about the client until after my visit with her is completed. I like to draw my own conclusions. This is a matter of personal preference. Having the consent form signed in your chart and asking permission to speak about her case with another practitioner are standard respectful and ethical practices.

There are ways to respectfully disagree with the advice attributed to other practitioners the mother has seen. You can say, "That practitioner made their best recommendation based on their experience and education. Based on my experience and education, I respectfully disagree." Following up with reasons why, offering a link to an article, or giving a copy of a relevant publication will support your practice. As a nurse, I was trained to never, ever disagree with a physician. However, the situation quickly arose where I knew far more about lactation than did the physician. Swallowing the truth for the sake of maintaining the power structure was neither pleasant nor healthy for me. Hence the collegial style of disagreement proposed here.

Time

Take enough time. When visits are scheduled and there is a limited amount of time allotted for each client, the practitioner's consciousness is diverted from paying full attention to the client a few minutes before the end of the visit. Once one begins to summarize, the energy changes directions and precious healing energy shifts away from the dyad.

Many times it takes an hour or more for the mother and baby to relax enough with each other in the office. This can be impedance to quick work. As babies are on their own schedules and can't be rushed, letting the dyad take its own time has proved effective.

I'm impressed with Chloe Fisher's breastfeeding clinic in Oxford, as seen in a video, where the room is full of nursing dyads, while the lactation staff moves from one to another. As women enjoy social networks, and nursing mothers' groups have been successful since 1956 (when La Leche League started), the notion of a breastfeeding therapist moving from one dyad to another is personally appealing. The therapist can work on baby time, instead of scheduling a visit and having to deal with a baby that may not want to feed. Centering Pregnancy™ is an example of successful group assessment, education, and support used for prenatal education (Centering Healthcare Institute, 2009). This is a solution to a busy schedule and could be used in lactation practice. Mothers can receive both individual attention and social support, and the therapist's time and energy can be used efficiently.

There seems to be a natural limit to the length of a visit. The range is between one and three hours. There are no working clocks in my office, and I don't wear a watch. From the thousands of pulses I have counted, I have an internal sense of the passage of seconds; that skill helps me in my assessments. Letting the dyad set the pace is freeing, delightfully effective, and feels right.

The length of time a mother and breastfeeding helper stays in contact can be flexible. After the first visit, a dyad may require daily contact. It is helpful to ask the mother "when do you want me to call you again?" One memorable teen wanted a telephone call every day for the first month; after a week or so, the calls were less than one minute long. "Hi Tanisha, how's it going?" "Fine." "Is Leonardo making lots of yellow poops?" "Yes."

"Are you having fun?" "Yes." "When do you want me to call you again?" "Tomorrow." After 30 telephone contacts, she felt confident to go solo. Many mothers have Internet access, and emails are another convenient way to stay in touch, with the advantage that there is a complete record of the dialogue. Once a mother is feeling in charge, the contacts dwindle away.

Confident mothers quickly seize the reins. Applaud their confidence, while leaving the door open to further interaction.

Summary

When I began my clinical career in lactation in 1975, there weren't many resources beyond La Leche League's brochures and fact sheets and their classic book, *The Womanly Art of Breastfeeding*. In 1986, there were only two breastfeeding videos available for parents, breastfeeding activists had an uphill battle to get hospitals to hire in-house lactation staff members, and the lactation consultant profession was one year old. The public was reluctant to spend money for lactation therapy, and no insurance companies would reimburse for lactation services. There was little available from public health or governmental agencies. Combining return to paid employment with breastfeeding was an individual struggle.

In 2011, the world has changed. The Internet is a major source of information and support through websites and chat rooms. The Centers for Disease Control provide information, conduct surveys, and share the results. The Department of Health and Human Services, the Surgeon General, and other governmental agencies are active sources of surveillance, statistics, and education; so is the U.S. Breastfeeding Committee. The Business Case for Breastfeeding is a well-designed, evidence-based strategy to help mothers in the workplace to sustain lactation. Breastfeeding rates and duration have increased since 1971. There is more to come.

At the same time, the formula industry is actively competing for the health of mothers and babies, using the Internet, marketing strategies, and flouting the International Code of Marketing of Breastmilk Substitutes to undermine women's confidence. This is manifested in the flat-line rates of breastfeeding exclusivity and duration for 2003-2007 (CDC, 2010f). Pump companies actively encourage human milk feeding, using many of the same strategies that have proved effective for the formula industry. A new cohort of women is choosing to pump and bottle-feed their milk instead of breastfeeding. Research has yet to reveal what impact this new trend will have on parenting and on health.

In the past 20 years, diabetes and obesity incidence and prevalence have become global epidemics, partly a consequence of insufficient breastfeeding. Estimates now are, if the trends are sustained, that babies born in the year 2000 will be the first generation with a shorter life expectancy than my generation (Belluck, 2005).

Diabetes, obesity, and environmental pollution are modern challenges to global health and life expectancy. These new challenges mean that now, more than ever, our babies need to breastfeed exclusively for about six months, to continue breastfeeding for one or two years as solid foods are gradually introduced, and to sustain the breastfeeding relationship for as long as mother and baby enjoy it (USDHHS, 2011; WHO, 2010).

Integrating complementary and alternative medicine and soft techniques are effective in restoring the connection between mother and baby, so breastfeeding lasts. Helping women to continue with breastfeeding who may have otherwise stopped is blessed and special work. I hope this book is useful and encourages lactation therapists, consultants, counselors, and breastfeeding helpers to add new tools to their toolboxes.

References

Academy of Breastfeeding Medicine (2011). Clinical protocols. Retrieved on January 11, 2011 from http://www.bfmed.org/Resources/Protocols.aspx.

Ahn, A.C., Wu, J., Badger, G.J., Hammerschlag, R., & Langevin, H.M. (2005). Electrical impedance along connective tissue planes associated with acupuncture meridians. *BMC Complementary and Alternative Medicine, 5*, 10.

Alcorn, K.L., O'Donovan, A., Patrick, J.C., Creedy, D., & Devilly, G.J. (2010). A prospective longitudinal study of the prevalence of post-traumatic stress disorder resulting from childbirth events. *Psychological Medicine, 40*(11), 1849-1859.

Alimi, D., Rubino, C., Pichard-Leandri, E., Fermand-Brule, S., Dubreuil-Lemaire, M.L., & Hill, C. (2003). Analgesic effect of auricular acupuncture for cancer pain: a randomized, blinded, controlled trial. *Journal of Clinical Oncology, 15, 21*(22), 4120-4126.

Althabe, F., & Belizan, J.M. (2006). Caesarean section: the paradox. *Lancet, 368*(9546), 1472-1473.

American Academy of Pediatrics. The use of complementary and alternative medicine in pediatrics. *Pediatrics, 122*(6), 1374- 1386.

AMA (American Medical Association). (1957). *Principles of medical ethics.* Retrieved February 21, 2011 from http://www.ama-assn.org/resources/doc/ethics/1957_principles.pdf.

AMA (American Medical Association). (1980). Principles of medical ethics. Retrieved March 30, 2011, from http://www.ama-assn.org/resources/doc/ethics/1980_principles.pdf.

AMA (American Medical Association). (1992). *AMA code of medical ethics. Opinion 3.041 – chiropractic.* Retrieved June 3, 2010 from http://www.ama-assn.org/ama/pub/physician-resources/medical-ethics/code-medical-ethics/opinion3041.shtml.

Aviner, S., Berkovitch, M., Dalkian, H., Braunstein, R., Lomnicky, Y., & Schlesinger, M. (2010). Use of a homeopathic preparation for "infantile colic" and an apparent life-threatening event. *Pediatrics, 125*(2), e318-e323.

Ayers, J.F. (2000). The use of alternative therapies in the support of breastfeeding. *Journal of Human Lactation, 16(1)*, 52-56.

Baby Friendly USA. (2010). *U.S. baby-friendly birth facilities.* Retrieved on February 27, 2011 from http://www.babyfriendlyusa.org/eng/03.html.

Barnes, P.M., Bloom, B., & Nahin, R.L. (2008). Complementary and alternative medicine use among adults and children: United States, 2007. *National Health Statistics Reports, 10*(12), 1–23.

Barr, R.G. (1999). Infant crying behavior and colic. In W. R. Trevathan, E.O. Smith, & J.J. McKenna (Eds.), *Evolutionary Medicine* (pp. 33-35). New York & Oxford: Oxford University Press.

Beck, C.T., & Watson, S. (2008). Impact of birth trauma on breastfeeding: a tale of two pathways. *Nursing Research, 57*(4), 228-236.

Belluck, P. (2005, March 17). Children's life expectancy being cut short by obesity. *New York Times*. Retrieved on February 27, 2011 from http://query.nytimes.com/gst/fullpage.html?res=9F01E3D7133CF934A25750C0A9639C8B63.

Bergman, N. (2011). What is KMC: Where it started. *Kangaroo Mother Care Promotions*. Accessed on April 25, 2011, from www.kangaroomothercare.com/whatis02.htm.

Blum, D. (2002). *Love at Goon Park* (p. 35). Jackson, TN: Perseus Publishing.

Bornhoft, G, Wolf, U., von Ammon, K. Righetti, M., Maxion-Bergemann, S., Baumgartner, S., et al. (2006). Effectiveness, safety, and cost-effectiveness of homeopathy in general practice--summarized health technology assessment. *Forschende Komplementarmedizin, 13(suppl 2)*, 19-29.

Bramson, L., Lee, J.W., Moore, E., Montgomery, S., Neish, C., Bahjri, K., et al. (2010). Effect of early skin-to-skin mother-infant contact during the first 3 hours following birth on exclusive breastfeeding during the maternity hospital stay. *Journal of Human Lactation, 26*, 130-137.

Brennan, B. (1993). *Light emerging: a journal of personal healing* (p. 31). New York: Bantam Books.

Cadwell, K., & Turner-Maffei, C. (2003). *Case studies in breastfeeding: problem-solving skills and strategies*. Sudbury, MA: Jones and Bartlett.

California State University (2011). *The orphanages*. Retrieved on December 26, 2009, from www.csuchico.edu/engl/faculty/engl1Tom/The%20Orphanages.html.

CDC (Centers for Disease Control). (2010a). *Breastfeeding among U.S. children born 1999-2007, CDC National Immunization Survey*. Retrieved on September 12, 2010 from www.CDC.gov/breastfeeding/data/NIS_data/index.htm.

CDC (Centers for Disease Control). (2010b). *2009 pediatric nutrition surveillance*. Retrieved on February 10, 2011 from http://www.cdc.gov/pednss/pednss_tables/pdf/national_table13.pdf.

CDC (Centers for Disease Control). (2010c). *2007 CDC national survey of maternity practices in infant nutrition and care (mPINC)*. Retrieved on September 5, 2010 from http://www.cdc.gov/breastfeeding/data/mpinc/index.htm.

CDC (Centers for Disease Control). (2010d). *NCHS data brief (35)*. Retrieved on February 10, 2011, from http://www.cdc.gov/nchs/data/databriefs/db35.htm.

CDC (Centers for Disease Control). (2010e). *Breastfeeding among U.S. children born 1999-2007, CDC national immunization survey*. Retrieved on February 10, 2011 from http://www.cdc.gov/breastfeeding/data/NIS_data/index.htm.

CDC (Centers for Disease Control). (2010f). *Data and statistics*. Retrieved on February 27, 2011 from http://www.cdc.gov/breastfeeding/data/index.htm.

Centering Healthcare Institute (2009). *Centering pregnancy overview*. Retrieved on February 27, 2011 from http://www.centeringhealthcare.org/pages/centering-model/pregnancy-overview.php.

Chapman, E.H. (1996). Letters to the editor: Homeopathic medicine. *Pediatrics, 97(5)*, 779.

Charpak, N., Ruiz, J.G., Zupan, J., Cattaneo, A., Figuero, Z., Tessier, R., et al. (2005). Kangaroo mother care: 25 years after. *Acta Paediatrica, 94(5)*, 514-22.

Chikly, B. (1999, August). *Lymph drainage therapy: Treatment for engorgement.* Presented at International Lactation Consultant Association Conference, Scottsdale, AZ. Audio tape: *Repeat Performance* 219-465-1234.

Chiropractic Resource Organization. (2010). *The Wilk case.* Retrieved May 23, 2010 from http://www.chiro.org/abstracts/amavschiro.pdf, p. 46.

Chiu, J.Y., Gau, M.L., Kuo, S.Y., Chang, Y.H., Kuo, S.C., & Tu, H.C. (2010). Effects of Gua-Sha therapy on breast engorgement: a randomized controlled trial. *Journal of Nursing Research, 18(1)*, 1-10.

Chiu, C.Y., Chang, C.Y., & Gau, M.L. (2008). An experience applying Gua-Sha to help a parturient women with breast fullness. *Hu Li Za Zhi, 55(1)*, 105-10.

Chiu, S.H., Anderson, G.C., & Burkhammer, M.D. (2008). Skin-to-skin contact for culturally diverse women having breastfeeding difficulties during early postpartum. *Breastfeeding Medicine, 3(4)*, 231-237.

Clavey, S. (1996). The use of acupuncture in the treatment of insufficient lactation (Que Ru). *American Journal of Acupuncture, 24*(1), 35-46.

Conde-Agudelo, A. & Belizán, J.M. (2003). *Kangaroo mother care to reduce morbidity and mortality in low birthweight infants.* Retrieved on December 6, 2010, from http://www2.cochrane.org/reviews/en/ab002771.html.

Colson, S. (2010). *An introduction to biological nurturing.* Amarillo, TX: Hale Publishing, p. 70.

Colson, S., Meek, H.H., & Hawdon, J.M. (2008). Optimal positions for the release of primitive neonatal reflexes stimulating breastfeeding. *Early Human Development, 84* (7) 441-449.

Cotterman, K.J. (2004). Reverse pressure softening: A simple tool to prepare areola for easier latching during engorgement. *Journal of Human Lactation, 20*, 227-237.

Coulton, G. (1906). *St. Francis to Dante.* London: David Nutt, pp. 242-43. Retrieved on June 14, 2010 from http://www.fordham.edu/halsall/source/salimbene1.html.

Creedy, D., Shochet, I.M., & Horsfall, J. (2001). Childbirth and the development of acute trauma symptoms: Incidence and contributing factors. *Birth, 27*(2), *104-111.*

Crivelli-Kovach, A., & Chung, E.K. (2010). An evaluation of hospital breastfeeding policies in the Philadelphia metropolitan area 1994-2009: A comparison with the Baby-Friendly Hospital Initiative Ten Steps. *Breastfeeding Medicine,* Epub ahead of print –Doi:10.1089/bfm.2010.009.

Damase-Michel, C., Vie, C., Lacroix, I., Lapeyre-Mestre, M., & Montastruc, J.L. (2004). Drug counselling in pregnancy: An opinion survey of French community pharmacists. *Pharmacoepidemiology and Drug Safety, 13*(10), 711-715.

de Araújo, C.L., Rios, C.T., dos Santos, M.H., & Goncalves, A.P. (2010). Mother kangaroo method: an investigation about the domestic practice. *Ciencia & Saude Coletiva, 15*(1), 301-307.

Dettwyler, K., & Stuart-Macadam, P. (Eds.). (1995). *Breastfeeding: biocultural perspectives*. Aldine Transaction, pp. 39-73.

Dewey, K.G., Nommsen-Rivers, L.A., Heinig, M.J., & Cohen, R.J. (2003). Risk factors for suboptimal infant breastfeeding behavior, delayed onset of lactation, and excess neonatal weight loss. *Pediatrics, 112*(3), 607-619.

Dickersin, K., & Mayer, M. (2009). understanding evidence-based healthcare: a foundation for action. U.S. Cochrane Centre online training course. Retrieved on March 15, 2011, from http://us.cochrane.org/understanding-evidence-based-healthcare-foundation-action.

Diego, M.A., Field, T., & Hernandez-Reif, M. (2005). Vagal activity, gastric motility and weight gain in massaged preterm neonates. *The Journal of Pediatrics, 147(1)*, 50-55.

Diego, M.A., Field, T., Hernandez-Reif, M., Deeds, O., Ascencio, A., & Begert, G. (2007). Preterm infant massage elicits consistent increases in vagal activity and gastric motility that are associated with greater weight gain. *Acta Pediatrica, 96* (11), 1588-1591.

Diego, M., Field T., Hernandez-Reif, M., Shaw, J.A., Rothe, E.M., Castellanos, D., & Mesner, L. (2002). Aggressive adolescents benefit from massage therapy. *Adolescence, 37*, 597-607.

Dieter, J.N., Field, T., Hernandez-Reif, M., Emory, E.K., & Redzepi, M. (2003). Stable preterm infants gain more weight and slept less after five days of massage therapy. *Journal of Pediatric Psychology, 28*(6), 403-411.

DiGirolamo, A.M., Grummer-Strawn, L.M., & Fein, S. (2001). Maternity care practices: implications for breastfeeding. *Birth, 28* (2), 94-100.

Dunbar, I. (2011). Handling & gentling. Adapted from *After you get your puppy*. Retrieved January 11, 2011 from http://www.dogstardaily.com/training/handling-and-gentling.

Ehrenreich, B., & English, D. (1973). *Witches, midwives, and healers*. Brooklyn, NY: The Feminist Press, p. 26.

Eisenberg, A., Murkoff, H.F., & Hathaway, S.E. (1996). *What to expect when you're expecting*. (2nd ed.) New York: Workman Publishing, p. 67.

Ernst, E., & Pittler, M.H. (1998). Efficacy of homeopathic arnica: A systematic review of placebo-controlled clinical trials. *Archives of Surgery, 133*(11), 1187-1190.

Evans, K.C., Evans, R.G., Royal, R., Esterman, A.J., & James, S.L. (2003). Effect of cesarean section on breast milk transfer to the normal term newborn over the first week of life. *Archives of Disease in Childhood. Fetal and Neonatal Edition*, 88(5), 380-388.

Fan, Y. (2004). *Chinese pediatric massage therapy*. Boulder, CO: Blue Poppy Press.

FDA. (1998). *FDA public health advisory: Need for CAUTION when using vacuum assisted delivery devices*. Retrieved on February 10, 2011, from www.fda.gov/MedicalDevices/Safety/AlertsandNotices/PublicHealthNotifications/UCM062295.

Ferber, S.G., Feldman, R., Kohelet, D.,Kuint, J., Dollberg, S., Arbel, E., et al. (2005). Massage therapy facilitates mother–infant interaction in premature infants. *Infant Behavior & Development, 28*(1), 74-81.

Field, T. (2010). Postpartum depression effects on early interactions, parenting, and safety practices: A review. *Infant Behavior & Development, 33*(1), 1-6.

Field, T. (Ed.). (2004). *Touch and massage in early child development.* Johnson & Johnson Pediatric Institute, pp. 115-136.

Field, T. (2002). Infants' need for touch. *Human Development, 157,* 1-4.

Field T., Diego, M., & Hernandez-Reif, M. (2010). Preterm infant massage therapy research: a review. *Infant Behavior & Development, 33(2),* 115-24.

Field, T., Diego, M., Hernandez-Reif, M., Dieter, J.N., Kumar, A.M., Schanberg, S., et al. (2008). Insulin and insulin-like growth factor-1 increased in preterm neonates following massage therapy. *Journal of Developmental & Behavioral Pediatrics, 29*(6), 463-466.

Field, T., Diego, M.A., Hernandez-Reif, M., Deeds, O., & Figuereido, B. (2006). Moderate versus light pressure massage therapy leads to greater weight gain in preterm infants. *Infant Behavior & Development, 29*(4), 574-578.

Field, T., Field, T., Cullen, C., Largie, S., Diego, M., Schanberg, S., et al. (2008). Lavender bath oil reduces stress and crying and enhances sleep in very young infants. *Early Human Development, 84*(6), 399-401.

Field, T.M., Schanberg, S.M., Scafidi, F., Bauer, C.R., Vega-Lahr, N., Garcia, R., et al. (1986). Tactile/kinesthetic stimulation effects on preterm neonates. *Pediatrics, 77*(5), 654-658.

Fisher, P., Dantas, F., & Reilly, D. (1996). Homeopathic treatment of childhood diarrhea. *Pediatrics, 97*(5), 776.

Flexner, A. (1910). *Medical education in the United States and Canada bulletin number four (The Flexner report).* Retrieved on January 25, 2011, from http://www.carnegiefoundation. org/publications/medical-education-united-states-and-canada-bulletin-number-four-flexner-report-0.

Foda, M.I., Kawashima, T., Nakamura, S., Kobayashi, M., & Oku, T. (2004). Composition of milk obtained from unmassaged versus massaged breasts of lactating mothers. *Journal of Pediatric Gastroenterology & Nutrition, 38*(5), 484-487.

Geddes, D.T. (2009). The use of ultrasound to identify milk ejection in women – tips and pitfalls. *International Breastfeeding Journal, 4,* 5.

Glover, R., & Wiessinger, D. (2008). The infant-maternal breastfeeding connection: Helping when they lose the thread. In C.W. Genna (Ed.). *Supporting sucking skills in breastfeeding infants* (pp. 97-128). Sudbury, MA: Jones and Bartlett Publishers.

Goer, H. (2007). *2007 CUE Summit.* Retrieved on January 13, 2011, from http://health. groups.yahoo.com/group/MFCInews/message/434.

Goldenberg, R.L., Culhane, J.F., Iams, J.D., & Romero, R. (2008). Epidemiology and causes of preterm birth. *Lancet, 371(9606),* 75-84.

Gooding, M.J., Finlay, J., Shipley, J.A., Halliwell, M., & Duck, F.A. (2010). Three-dimensional ultrasound imaging of mammary ducts in lactating women: A feasibility study. *Journal of Ultrasound in Medicine, 29*(1), 95-103.

Gori, L., & Firenzuoli, F. (2007). Ear acupuncture in European traditional medicine. *Evidence-based Complementary and Alternative Medicine, 4*(1), 13-16. Retrieved on February 15, 2011, from http://www.sedatelec.com/english/acupauri.htm.

Gouin, J.P., Kiecolt-Glaser, J.K., Malarkey, W.B., & Glaser, R. (2008). The influence of anger expression on wound healing. *Brain, Behavior, and Immunity, 22*(5), 699-708. Retrieved December 11, 2010, from www.uppitysciencechick.com.

Grajeda. R., & Perez-Escamilla, R. (2002). Stress during labor and delivery is associated with delayed onset of lactation among urban Guatemalan women. *Journal of Nutrition, 132(10)*, 3055-60.

Gregory, W.M., Mills, S.P., Hamed, H.H., & Fentiman, I.S. (2001). Applied kinesiology for treatment of women with mastalgia, *Breast, 10*(1), 15-19.

Green, C., Martin, C.W., Bassett, K., & Kazanjian, A. (1999). A systematic review of craniosacral therapy: biological plausibility, assessment reliability and clinical effectiveness. *Complementary Therapies in Medicine, 7*(4), 201-207.

Grummer-Strawn, L.M., Scanlon, K.S., & Fein, S.B. (2008). Infant feeding and feeding transitions during the first year of life. *Pediatrics, 122*(Supp 2), S36-S42.

Harlow, H. (1958). The nature of love. *American Psychologist, 13*, 673-685.

Harding, D., & Foureur, M. (2009). New Zealand and Canadian midwives' use of complementary and alternative medicine. *New Zealand College of Midwives Journal, 40*, 7-12.

Harris H. (1994). Remedial co-bathing for breastfeeding difficulties. *Breastfeeding Reviews, 11*(10), 465-468.

Henry, J. (1987) Medicine and pneumatology: Henry More, Richard Baxter, and Francis Glisson's Treatise on the Energetic Nature of Substance. *Medical History, 31*(1), 15-40.

Hoddinott, P., Britten, J., & Pill, R. (2010). Why do interventions work in some places and not others: A breastfeeding support group trial. *Social Science & Medicine, 70*, 774.

Holla, M., Ijland, M.M., Verlaat, C.W.M., van der Vliet, A.M., & Edwards, M. (2009). Infant dies after "craniosacral" therapy. *Ned Tijdschr Geneeskd, 153*, A290. Retrieved on January 13, 2011, from http://anaximperator.wordpress.com/2009/05/07/infant-dies-after-craniosacral-therapy/.

Holson, L. (2005, April 25). The feng shui kingdom. *The New York Times*. Retrieved on January 25, 2011 from http://query.nytimes.com/gst/fullpage.html?res=9A00E6D8 1531F936A15757C0A9639C8B63&sec=&spon=&pagewanted=1.

Hurst, N.M., Valentine, C.J., Renfro, L., Burns, P., & Ferlic, L. (1997). Skin-to-skin holding in the neonatal intensive care unit influence maternal milk volume. *Journal of Perinatology,17*(3), 213-217.

IBCLE (International Board of Lactation Consultant Examiners). (2008). *Scope of practice for International Board Certified Lactation Consultants*. Retrieved on April 8, 2010, from http://www.iblce.org/upload/downloads/ScopeOfPractice.pdf.

Jacobs, J., Jimenez, L.M., Gloyd, S.S., Gale, J.L., & Crothers, D. (1996). Letter to the editor. *Pediatrics, 97(5)*, 778-779.

Jacobs, J., Jimenez, L.M., Gloyd, S.S., Gale, J.L., & Crothers, D. (1994). Treatment of acute childhood diarrhea with homeopathic medicine: a randomized clinical trial in Nicaragua. *Pediatrics, 93*(5), 719-725.

Jenner, C., & Filshie, J. (2002). Galactorrhoea following acupuncture. *Acupuncture in Medicine, 20*(2-3), 107-108.

Joswick, D. (2011). *Historic points: Acupuncture needles*. Retrieved on January 25, 2011, from http://www.acufinder.com/Acupuncture+Information/Detail/Historic+Points+Ac upuncture+Needles.

Karl, D.J. (2004). Using principles of newborn behavioral state organization to facilitate breastfeeding. *The American Journal of Maternal Child Nursing, 29*(5), 292-298.

Kato, K., Nagata, I., Furuya, K., Seki, IK., & Makimura, N. (1994). Programmed induction of labor for primiparous women to ensure daytime delivery. *Asia-Oceania Journal of Obstetrics and Gynecology, 13*(4), 405-415.

Kemper, K.J., Vohra, S., Walls, R., Task Force on Complementary and Alternative Medicine, Provisional Section on Complementary, Holistic, and Integrative Medicine. (2008). American Academy of Pediatrics. The use of complementary and alternative medicine in pediatrics. *Pediatrics, 122*(6), 1374-1386.

Kennell, J.H., & Klaus, M.H. (1998). Bonding: Recent observations that alter prenatal care. *Pediatrics in Review, 19*(1), 4-12.

Kennell, J.H., Trause, M.A., & Klaus, M.H. (1975). Evidence for a sensitive period in the human mother. *Ciba Foundation Symp*osium*, 33*, 87-101.

Kirchner, A., Birklein, F., Stefan, H., & Handwerker, H.O. (2000). Left vagus nerve stimulation suppresses experimentally induced pain. *Neurology, 55*(8), 1167-1171.

Klaus, M.H., Trause, M.A., & Kennell, J.H. (1975). Does human material behavior after delivery show a characteristic pattern? *Ciba Foundation Symposium,* (33), 69-85.

Klaus, M.H., & Kennell, J.H. (1982). *Parent-infant bonding*. St. Louise: Mosby, Chapter 4.

Klaus, M.H., Kennell, J.H., & Klaus, P.H. (1995). *Bonding*. Reading, MA: Addison-Wesley Publishing Co, Inc, pp. 57-59.

Klaus, M.H. & Klaus, P.H. (1985). *The amazing newborn*. Reading, MA: Addison-Wesley Publishing Co., p. 53.

Kornfield, J., & Feldman, C. (1996). *Soul food. Stories to nurture the spirit and the heart*. New York: Harper Collins, p. 115.

Kundtz, D. (1998). *Stopping: How to be still when you have to keep going*. Newburyport, MA: Conari Press.

Kvist, L.J., Hall-Lord, M.L., Rydhstroem, H., Larsson, B.W. (2007). A randomized-controlled trial in Sweden of acupuncture and care interventions for relief of inflammatory symptoms of the breast during lactation. *Midwifery, 23*(2), 184-195.

Lahat, S., Mimouni, F.B., Ashbel, G., & Dollberg, S. (2007). Energy expenditure in growing preterm infants receiving massage therapy. *Journal of the American College of Nutrition, 26*(4), 356-359.

Lämås, K., Lindholm, L., Stenlund, H., Engstrom, B., & Jacobsson, C. (2009). Effects of abdominal massage in management of constipation--A randomized controlled trial. *International Journal of Nursing Studies, 46*(6), 759-767.

Lawrence, R.A. (1994). *Breastfeeding: A guide for the medical profession* (4th Ed.) St. Louis: Mosby, p. 243.

Lee, H.K. (2006). The effects of infant massage on weight, height, and mother-infant interaction. *Taehan Kanho Hakhoe Chi,36*(8), 1331-9.

Lee, N. (2005). Cycle of seeking, emotional outburst, and rest in newborns put to the breast. *Journal of Human Lactation, 21*(2), 120.

Lee, N. (1997). Observations based upon multiple telephone contacts with new breastfeeding mothers. *Journal of Human Lactation, 13*(2), 147- 150.

Leung, G.M. (2000). Hospitals must become focused factories. *BMJ, 320*(7239), 942-943.

Li, K. (2003). A pilot study to evaluate the effect of acupuncture on increasing milk supply of lactating mothers. Master's thesis: Victoria University. Retrieved on February 11, 2011 from http://wallaby.vu.edu.au/adt-VVUT/public/adt-VVUT20031203.093949/.

Lockie, A. (1989). *The family guide to homeopathy* (p. 1). Palmer, AK: Fireside Books.

Lu, P., Qiu, J., Yao, F., & Zheng, J.J. (2010). Effect of acupoint Tuina on lactation amount for parturient. *Zhongguo Ahen Jiu, 30*(9), 731-733.

Lubetsky, R., Littner, Y., Mimouni, F.B., Dollberg, S., & Mandel, D. (2006). Circadian variations in fat content of expressed breast milk of mothers of preterm infants. *Journal of the American College of Nutrition, 25*(2), 151-154.

Ludtke, R., Kunz, B., Seeber, N., & Ring, J. (2001) Test-rest-reliability and validity of kinesiology muscle test. *Complementary Therapies in Medicine, 9*(3), 141-145.

Lund, G.C., Edwards, G., Medlin, B., Keller, D., Beck, B., & Carreiro, J.E. (2011). Osteopathic manipulative treatment for the treatment of hospitalized premature infants with nipple feeding dysfunction. *The Journal of the American Osteopathic Association, 111*(1), 44-48.

Lvoff, N.M., Lvoff, V., & Klaus, M.H. (2000). Effect of the baby-friendly initiative on infant abandonment in a Russian hospital. Archives of Pediatric and Adolescent Medicine, 154(5), 474-477.

MacDorman, M.F., Declercq, E., & Zhang, J. (2010). Obstetrical intervention and the singleton preterm birth rate in the United States. *American Journal of Public Health, 100*(11), 2241-2247.

Madrid, A., & Pennington, D. (2000). Maternal-infant bonding and asthma. *Journal of Prenatal and Perinatal Psychology and Health, 14*(3-4). Retrieved on January 11, 2011 from http://www.rivershrink.com/study.html.

Mangesi, L. & Dowswell, T. (2011). Treatments for breast engorgement during lactation. *Cochrane Database of Systematic Reviews 2010*, Issue 9. Retrieved on February 10, 2011 from http://www2.cochrane.org/reviews/en/ab006946.html.

Massage London. (2011). Breast massage treatment to reduce breasts pain. Retrieved on January 11, 2011 from http://massagelondon.org/pages/brstmsg.htm.

Mathie, R.T. (2003). The research evidence base for homeopathy: a fresh assessment of the literature. *Homeopathy, 92*(2), 84-91.

Matthieson, A.S., Ransjo-Arvidson, A.B., Nissen, E., & Uvnas-Moberg, K. (2001). Postpartum maternal oxytocin release by newborns: effects of infant hand massage and sucking. *Birth, 28*(1), 13-19.

Mayer, D. (2000). Acupuncture: an evidence-based review of the clinical literature. *Annual Review of Medicine, 51,* 49-63. Retrieved on February 11, 2011, from http://ukpmc.ac.uk/abstract/MED/10774452/reload=0;jsessionid=BCECA1EDCED3BF02D7C998E712E06A8F.jvm1.

McCallister, H., Bradshaw, S., & Ross-Adjie, G. (2009). A study of in-hospital midwifery practices that affect breastfeeding outcomes. *Breastfeeding Review, 17*(3), 11-15.

Mechanic, D., McAlpine, D.D., & Rosenthal, M.A. (2001). Are patients' office visits with physicians getting shorter? *New England Journal of Medicine, 344*, 198-204. Retrieved on February 10, 2011 from http://content.nejm.org/cgi/content/full/344/3/198/F1.

Mendes, E. W., & Procianoy, R.S. (2008). Massage therapy reduces hospital stay and occurrence of late-onset sepsis in very preterm neonates. *Journal of Perinatology, 28*(12), 815-820.

Merrell, W.C., & Shalts, E. (2002). Homeopathy. *The Medical Clinics of North America, 86(1)*, 47-62.

Meyer, K., & Anderson, G.C. (1999). Using kangaroo care in a clinical setting with full-term infants having breastfeeding difficulties. *MCN. The American Journal of Maternal Child Nursing, 24*(4), 190-192.

Mikiel-Kostyra, K., Mazur, J., & Boltruszko, I. (2002). Effect of early skin-to-skin contact after delivery on duration of breastfeeding: a prospective cohort study. *Acta Paediatrica, 91*(12), 1301-1306.

Miller, V., & Riordan, J. (2004). Treating postpartum breast edema with areolar compression. *Journal of Human Lactation, 20*(2), 223-226.

Miller, J.E., Miller, L., Sulesund, A.K., & Yevtushenko, A. (2009). Contribution of chiropractic therapy to resolving suboptimal breastfeeding: a case series of 114 infants. *Journal of Manipulative and Physiological Therapeutics, 32*(8), 670-674.

Moncayo, R., Moncayo, H., Ulmer, H., & Kainz, H. (2004). New diagnostic and therapeutic approach to thyroid-associated orbitopathy based on applied kinesiology and homeopathic therapy. *Journal of Alternative and Complementary Medicine, 10*(4), 643-650.

Montague (1986). *Touching: The human significance of skin* (3rd ed.). New York: Harper & Row, p. 4.

Moore, E.R., & Anderson, G.C. (2007). Randomized controlled trial of very early mother-infant skin-to-skin contact and breastfeeding status. *Journal of Midwifery & Women's Health, 52*(2), 116-125.

Moore, E.R., Anderson, G.C., & Bergman, N. (2007). Early skin-to-skin contact for mothers and their healthy newborn infants. *Cochrane Database of Systematic Reviews, 3*, CD003519. Retrieved on March 21, 2010 from http://mrw.interscience.wiley.com/cochrane/clsysrev/articles/CD003519/frame.html.

Morrison, B., Ludington-Hoe, S., & Anderson, G.C. (2006). Interruptions to breastfeeding dyads on postpartum day 1 in a university hospital. *Journal of Obstetric, Gynecologic, and Neonatal Nursing, 35*(6), 709-716.

Morrel, P. (2011). *A brief biography of Samuel Hahnemann.* Retrieved on February 27, 2011, from http://www.heilkunst.com/biography.html.

Morton, J., Hall, J.Y., Wong, R.J., Thairu, L., Benitz, W.E., & Rhine, W.D. (2009). Combining hand techniques with electric pumping increases milk production in mothers of preterm infants. *Journal of Perinatology, 29*(11), 757–764.

Moyer-Mileur, L.J., Ball, S.D., Brunstetter, V.L., & Chan, G.M. (2008). Maternal-administered physical activity enhances bone mineral acquisition in premature very low birth weight infants. *Journal of Perinatology, 28*(6), 432-437.

Nahin, R.L., Barnes, P.M., Stussman, B.J., & Bloom, B. (2009). Costs of complementary and alternative medicine (CAM) and frequency of visits to CAM practitioners: United States, 2007. *National Health Statistics Reports, (18), 1-14.*

Nayak, S., Matheis, R.J., Schoenberger, N.E., & Shiflett, S.C. (2003). Use of unconventional therapies by individuals with multiple sclerosis. *Clinical Rehabilitation, 17*(2), 181-191.

NCCAM (National Center for Complementary and Alternative Medicine). (2010). Chiropractic: An introduction. *National Institutes of Health.* Retrieved January 11, 2011 from http://nccam.nih.gov/health/chiropractic/introduction.htm.

NCCAM (National Center for Complementary and Alternative Medicine). (2009). Spinal manipulation for low-back pain. *National Institutes of Health.* Retrieved August 21, 2010 from http://nccam.nih.gov/health/pain/D409_GTF.pdf.

Niala, C. (2010). *Why African babies don't cry: An African perspective.* Retrieved on September 18, 2010, from http://www.naturalchild.org/guest/claire_niala.html.

NIH (National Institutes of Health). (1997). Acupuncture. *NIH Consensus Statement, 15*(5), 1-34.

Nissen, E., Uvnas-Moberg, K., Svensson, K., Stock, S., Widstrom, A.M., & Winberg, J. (1996). Different patterns of oxytocin, prolactin but not cortisol release during breastfeeding in women delivered by caesarean section or by the vaginal route. *Early Human Development,45*(1-2), 103-118.

Nommsen-Rivers, L.A., & Dewey, K.G. (2009). Growth of breastfed infants. *Breastfeeding Medicine, 4*(1), S45-S49.

Odent, M. (1999). *The scientification of love* (pp. 6-8). London: Free Association Books.

O'Higgins, M., St James Roberts, I., & Glover, V. (2008). Postnatal depression and mother and infant outcomes after infant massage. *Journal of Affective Disorders, 109*(1-2), 189-192.

Olafsdottir, E., Forshei, S., Fluge, G., & Markestad, T. (2001). Randomised controlled trial of infantile colic treated with chiropractic spinal manipulation, *Archives of Disease in Childhood, 84*(2), 138-141.

Onozawa, K., Glover, V., Adams, D., Modi, N., & Kumar, R.C. (2001). Infant massage improves mother-infant interaction for mothers with postnatal depression. *Journal of Affective Disorders, 63*(1-3), 201-207.

OSHA (Occupational Safety & Health Administration). (1996). *Presenting effective presentations with visual aids.* Retrieved on February 10, 2011, from www.osha.gov/doc/outreachtraining/htmlfiles/traintec.html.

Osler, W. (1860). Currents and counter-currents in medical science. Address to Massachusetts Medical Society (May 30, 1860). In O. W. Holmes, *Medical Essays 1842-1882* (1891), 202-3.

Parker-Pope, T. (2011). *Nutrition advice from the China Study.* Retrieved February 10, 2011 from http://well.blogs.nytimes.com/2011/01/07/nutrition-advice-from-the-china-study/?src=me&ref=health.

Pattinson, R.C., Bergh, A.M., Malan, A.F., & Prinsloo, R. (2006). Does kangaroo mother care save lives? *Journal of Tropical Pediatrics, 52*(6), 438-441.

Pennicott, K. (2001). *Lasers illuminate the flight of the bumblebee.* Retrieved on January 13, 2011, from http://physicsworld.com/cws/article/news/3410.

Philipp, B.L., Merewood, A., Miller, L.W., Chawla, N., Murphy-Smith, M.M., Gomes, J.S., et al. (2001). Baby-Friendly Hospital Initiative improves breastfeeding initiation rates in a U.S. hospital setting. *Pediatrics, 108*(3), 677-681.

Pothmann, R., von Frankenberg, S., Hoicke, C., Weingarten, H., & Ludtke, R. (2001). Evaluation of applied kinesiology in nutritional intolerance of childhood. *Forschende Komplementarmedzin und Klassiche Naturheilkunde, 8*(6), 336-344.

Pernick (1987). *Why infant surgery without anesthesia went unchallenged.* Retrieved on December 31, 2010 from http://www.nytimes.com/1987/12/17/opinion/l-why-infant-surgery-without-anesthesia-went-unchallenged-124987.html.

Puig, G, and Sguassero Y. (2007). *Early skin-to-skin contact for mothers and their healthy newborn infants: RHL commentary.* Retrieved on March 23, 2011, from http://apps.who.int/rhl/newborn/gpcom/en/index.html.

Ramchandani, N.M. (2010). Homoeopathic treatment of upper respiratory tract infections in children: evaluation of thirty case series. *Complementary Therapies in Clinical Practice, 16*(2), 101-108.

Ramsay, D.T., Kent, J.C., Hartmann, R.A., & Hartmann, P.E. (2005). Anatomy of the lactating human breast redefined with ultrasound imaging. *Journal of Anatomy, 206*(6), 525-534.

Razvi, S., Ingoe, L.E., McMillan, C.V., & Weaver, J.U. (2005). Health status in patients with sub-clinical hypothyroidism. *European Journal of Endocrinology, 152*(5), 713-717.

Remen, N.R. (1996). *Kitchen table wisdom.* New York: Riverhead Books, p. 239.

Reyna, B.A., & Pickler, R.H. (2009). Mother-infant synchrony. *Journal of Obstetrics, Gynecologic, and Neonatal Nursing, 38*(4), 470-478.

Richmond, R.L. (2011). *A guide to psychology and its practice.* Retrieved on February 10, 2011, from http://www.guidetopsychology.com/stress.htm.

Righard, L., & Alade, M.O. (1990). Effect of delivery room routines on success of first breast-feed. *Lancet, 336*(8723), 1105-1107.

Rogoff, B. (2003). *The cultural nature of human development.* p. 64. USA: Oxford University Press.

Rowe-Murray, H.J., & Fisher, J.R. (2001). Operative intervention in delivery is associated with compromised early mother-infant interaction. *BJOG, 108*(10), 1068-75.

Ruiz-Pelaez, J.G., Charpak, N., & Cuervo, L.G. (2004). Kangaroo Mother Care, an example to follow from developing countries. *BMJ, 329*(7475), 1179-1181.

Sackett, D.L. (1997). Evidence-based medicine. *Seminars in Perinatology, 21*(1), 3-5.

Sakala, C., & Corry, M.P. (2008). *Evidence-based maternity care: What it is and what it can achieve.* Retrieved on February 10, 2011 from http://www.milbank.org/reports/0809Materni tyCare/0809MaternityCare.html.

Saraswat, P. (1998). *A historical perspective on the philosophical foundations of information systems.* Retrieved on February 10, 2011 from http://www.bauer.uh.edu/parks/fis/saraswat3. htm.

Schlitz, M.J., & LaBerge, S. (1997). Covert observation increases skin conductance in subjects unaware of when they are being observed: A replication. *Journal of Parapsychology, 61*, 187-196.

Schnyer, R., Lao, L., Hammerschlag, R., Wayne, P., Langevin, H.M., Napadow, V., Harris, R., et al. (2008). Society for Acupuncture Research: 2007 conference report: The status and future of acupuncture research: 10 years post–NIH Consensus Conference. *Journal of Alternative and Complementary Medicine, 14*(7), 859-860.

Serrano, M.S., Doren, F.M., & Wilson, L. (2010). Teaching Chilean mothers to massage their full-term infants: effects on maternal breastfeeding and infant weight gain at age 2 and 4 months. *The Journal of Perinatal & Neonatal Nursing, 24*(2), 172-181.

Shin, H.S., Song, Y.A., & Seo, S. (2007). Effect of Nei-Guan point (P6) acupressure on ketonuria levels, nausea and vomiting in women with hyperemesis gravidarium. *Journal of Advanced Nursing, 59*(5), 510-519.

Simkin, P. (1991). Just another day in a woman's life? Women's long-term perceptions of their first birth experience. Part 1. *Birth, 18*(4), 203-210.

Sinusas, K., & Gagliardi, A. (2001). Initial management of breastfeeding. *American Family Physician, 64*(6), 981-988.

Smith, L. (2010). *The impact of birthing practices on breastfeeding* (2nd Ed.). Sudbury, MA: Jones and Bartlett.

Sosa, R., Kennell, J., Klaus, M., Robertson, S., & Urrutia, J. (1980). The effect of a supportive companion on perinatal problems, length of labor, and mother-infant interaction. *New England Journal of Medicine, 303*(11), 597-600.

Sotiriadis, A., Makrydimas, G., Papatheodorou, S., & Ioannidis, J.P. (2009). Corticosteroids for preventing neonatal respiratory morbidity after elective caesarean section at term. *Cochrane Database of Systematic Reviews, 7*(4):CD006614.

Starfield, B. (2000). Is US health really the best in the world? *JAMA 284*(4), 483-485.

Stern, D. (1998). *The birth of a mother* (pp. 93-109). New York: Basic Books.

Stutte, P.C., Bowles, B.C., & Morman, G.Y. (1988). The effects of breast massage on volume and fat content of human milk. *Genesis, 10*, 22-25.

Sugarman, M., & Kendall-Tackett, K.A. (1995). Weaning ages in a sample of American women who practice extended breastfeeding. *Clinical Pediatrics, 34*(12), 642-647.

Taylor, J.B. (2006). *My stroke of insight* (p. 18). New York: Penguin Group.

Teuber, S.S., & Porch-Curren, C. (2003) Unproved diagnostic and therapeutic approaches to food allergy and intolerance. *Current Opinion in Allergy & Clinical Immunology, 3*(3), 217-221.

Thomason, S. (2003). An early language experiment: Failure or triumph? Retrieved on June 13, 2010, from http://itre.cis.upenn.edu/~myl/languagelog/archives/000078.html.

Turner, R.A., Altemus, M., Enos, T., Cooper, B., & McGuinness, T. (1999). Preliminary research on plasma oxytocin in normal cycling women: investigating emotion and interpersonal distress. *Psychiatry, 62*(2), 97-113.

Upledger, J. (2005). *Working wonders* (p. XV). Berkeley, CA: North Atlantic Books.

Upledger, J. (1997). *Your inner physician and you* (pp. 9-14). Berkeley, CA: North Atlantic Books.

Uvnäs Moberg, K. (2003). *The oxytocin factor* (pp. 135-141). Cambridge, MA: Da Capo Press.

USDHHS (U.S. Dept. of Health and Human Services). (2011). *Maternal, infant and child health. Healthy People 2020 objectives.* Retrieved on February 27, 2011 from http://www.healthypeople.gov/2020/topicsobjectives2020/objectiveslist.aspx?topicid=26.

USDHHS (U.S. Dept. of Health and Human Services). (2010). Births: Final data for 2008. *National Vital Statistics Reports, 59(1).* Retrieved on February 13, 2011 from http://suporior-surrogacy.com/nchs/data/nvsr/nvsr59/nvsr59_01.pdf.

USDHHS (U.S. Dept. of Health and Human Services). (2009a). Births: Preliminary Data for 2007. *National Vital Statistics Reports, 57(12).* Retrieved on February 10, 2011 from http://www.cdc.gov/nchs/data/nvsr/nvsr57/nvsr57_12.pdf?loc=interstitialskip.

Vallone, S.A. (2004). Chiropractic care for the breastfeeding dyad. *Leaven, 39*(6), 126-127. Retrieved January 11, 2011 from http://www.llli.org/llleaderweb/LV/LVDecJan04p126.html.

Van Teijlingen, E., Porter, M., Lowis, G.W., & McCaffery, P.G. (Eds.). (2004). *Midwifery and the medicalization of childbirth: Comparative perspectives* (p. 107). Hauppauge, NY: Nova Publishers.

Verny, T., & Kelly, J. (1982). *The secret life of the unborn child: How you can prepare your baby for a happy, healthy life* (p. 36-38). New York: Dell Publishing.

Vignochi, C.M., Miura, E., & Canani, L.H. (2008). Effects of motor physical therapy on bone mineralization in premature infants: A randomized controlled study. *Journal of Perinatology, 28* (9), 624-631.

Von Knorring, A.L., Soderberg, A., Austin, L., & Uvnäs-Moberg, K. (2008). Massage decreases aggression in pre-school children: A long-term study. *Acta Pediatrica, 97*(9), 1265-1269.

Walker, M. (2000). Breastfeeding and engorgement. *Breastfeeding Abstracts, 20*(2), 11-12. Retrieved on March 23, 2011 from http://www.llli.org/ba/Nov00.html.

Wall, V., & Glass, R. (2006). Mandibular asymmetry and breastfeeding problems: Experience from 11 cases. *Journal of Human Lactation, 22*(3), 328-334.

Whitelaw, W.A. (2002). The historical development of chiropractic (p. 58). *The Proceedings of the 11th Annual History of Medicine Days.* Retrieved on May 23, 2010, from http://www.ucalgary.ca/uofc/Others/HOM/Dayspapers2002.pdf.

Widstrom, A.M., Lilja, G., Aaltomaa-Michalias, P., Dahllof, A., Lintula, M., & Nissen, E. (2011). Newborn behavior to locate the breast when skin-to-skin: A possible method for enabling early self-regulation. *Acta Paediatrica 100*(1), 79-85.

Widstrom, A.M., Wahlberg, V., Matthiesen, A.S., Eneroth, P., Uvnas-Moberg, K., Werner, S., et al. (1990). Short-tem effects of early suckling and touch of the nipple on maternal behavior. *Early Human Development, 21*(3), 153-163.

Wiessinger, D. (2009, July). *Everything old is new again.* Presented at the La Leche League International meeting, Philadelphia, Pennsylvania.

Wilkinson, D. (1998). *Bumblebees flying.* Retrieved on January 13, 2011, from http://www.math.niu.edu/~rusin/known-math/98/bees.

Wilson-Clay, B., & Hoover, K. (2008). *The breastfeeding atlas* (3rd ed., pp. 111). Austin, TX: LactNews Press.

WHO (World Health Organization). (2011). *Breastfeeding counselling: A training course.* Retrieved on February 27, 2011, from http://www.who.int/child_adolescent_health/documents/pdfs/bc_participants_manual.pdf.

WHO (World Health Organization). (2010). *Outline of a comprehensive implementation plan on infant and young child nutrition as a critical component of a global multisectoral nutrition framework.* Retrieved on February 27, 2011, from http://www.who.int/nutrition/EB128_18_Nutrition_CIP_outline.pdf.

WHO (World Health Organization), & UNICEF (2009). *Home visits for the newborn child: a strategy to improve survival.* Retrieved on March 21, 2010, from www.who.int/child_adolescent_health/documents/who_fch_cah_09_02.

World Health Organization. (1998). *Evidence for the Ten Steps to Successful Breastfeeding* (p. 31). Geneva: World Health Organization.

WHO (World Health Organization). (1985). Appropriate technology for birth. *Lancet, 2*(9452), 436-437.

Yellott, G. (2001). The loving touch: More than just a therapy. *J Neonatal Nursing, 7(6)*, 207-208.

Zhang, J., Liu, Y., Meikle, S., Zheng, J., Sun, W., & Li, Z. (2008). Cesarean delivery on maternal request in Southeast China. *Obstetrics & Gynecology, 111*(5), 1077-82.

Index

Author Bio

Nikki Lee has been a passionate advocate for the mother-infant relationship since the birth of her first daughter in 1975. This passion was re-dedicated in 1990 with the birth of her second daughter. Her career encompasses teaching, clinical practice, writing, public speaking, and research.

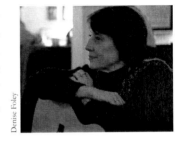

Denise Foley

Nikki's clinical practice includes work as a childbirth educator, a craniosacral therapy practitioner, an infant massage instructor, a lactation consultant, and a registered nurse. Her personal joy and renewal comes from playing music (back-up guitar in Cajun, Irish and Old-time styles, and bodhran), figure skating (currently working on silver moves in the field), dancing, hiking, and spiritual growth.

Nikki dreams of the day when war and polluting practices are abandoned because they are not good for babies, and where everyone everywhere works for clean air, clean Earth, and clean water, so our precious babies have healthy lives.

Ordering Information

Hale Publishing, L.P.
1712 N. Forest Street
Amarillo, Texas, USA 79106

8:00 am to 5:00 pm CST

Call » 806.376.9900
Toll free » 800.378.1317
Fax » 806.376.9901

Online Orders
www.ibreastfeeding.com